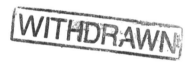

Asthma:
ASK THE
Experts

Asthma:
ASK THE
Experts

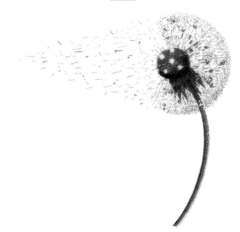

National Asthma
Training Centre

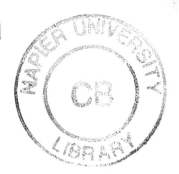

CLASS PUBLISHING · LONDON

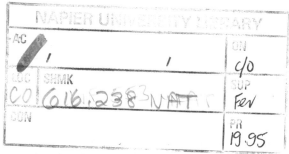

© National Asthma Training Centre 1997

Printing history
First published 1997

The authors and the publishers welcome feedback from the users of this book. Please contact the publishers.
Class Publishing (London) Ltd, Barb House, Barb Mews, London W6 7PA
Telephone: 0171 371 2119
Fax: 0171 371 2878 [International +44171]

A CIP catalogue record for this book is available from the British Library

ISBN 1 872362 68 0

Designed by Wendy Bann

Edited by Ruth Midgley

Back cover photograph by Greta Barnes

Produced by Landmark Production Consultants Ltd, Princes Risborough

Typesetting by DP Photosetting, Aylesbury, Bucks

Printed and bound in Slovenia by printing house Delo Tiskarna by arrangement with Korotan Ljubljana

Foreword

Professor T.J.H. Clark, MD, BSc, FRCP,
Dean and Professor of Pulmonary Medicine at the National Heart and Lung Institute, Imperial College of Science, Technology and Medicine, London and Consultant Physician at the Royal Brompton Hospital, London.

The growing burden of asthma has been accompanied by increasing knowledge about its cause and treatment. Much expenditure of time, effort and money has been devoted to research into the causes of asthma, and to developing new treatments as well as improvements in the diagnosis and assessment of asthma. The added value of this increase in knowledge has been considerable but it needs to be harnessed by patients and those who care for them. Knowledge without application is of marginal value to those with asthma, who suffer as individuals from this disease, and to society, which increasingly bears the growing financial burden.

The National Asthma Training Centre has provided a much needed bridge between our knowledge of asthma and its application. It has been largely responsible for the considerable improvement in patient care. Its impact has been enormous, with cadres of its trainees carrying knowledge and its application into primary care throughout the country. The network of Trainers and Instructors has supervised the delivery, by nurses working in general practice, of knowledge and experience which has been codified as guidelines. Guidelines are not rules but advice from experts, which require messengers with skill to transmit the information and guidance to the individual patient. All of us act as messengers with varying degrees of success, but a well trained person in primary care brings the message direct to the patient and is particularly effective.

The seminal role of the National Asthma Training Centre in our attempts to improve asthma care ensured that all the experts willingly gave their time to produce this personalised synopsis. This new initiative should further help in the task of informing patients and aiding them to apply the knowledge recently acquired and summarised by the experts.

This book is thus a testimonial from all the experts to the enormous good that has come from the National Asthma Training Centre; Greta Barnes and her team have done wonders for asthma and this is our tribute.

v

Contents

Chapter 5 Asthma Education: For patients and professionals

Introduction

Greta Barnes, MBE, SRN,
Director, National Asthma Training Centre

This book is for any health professional, particularly doctors and specialist asthma nurses, who manage patients suffering from asthma.

For many of these health professionals it is often the personal view of an expert that is of interest and value. This book has been developed to reflect the wealth of knowledge which many experts have gained through their experience, research and interest in the field of asthma. It has not been designed to fulfil the role of a text book or to be a practical guide for the management of asthma. Instead, over 100 experts have been invited to contribute answers to important questions about asthma and other related conditions. Hence the title "**Asthma: Ask the Experts**".

Each contributor has answered a question from an area in which he or she is considered to be an acknowledged authority. There are quite deliberately no footnotes or references and each author has been encouraged to give his or her own personal view.

Whilst there is general agreement that asthma care has improved significantly over the last 10 years there is no room for complacency. The condition continues to cause a high level of morbidity and economic burden as well as substantial, often unnecessary, mortality. The number of people who have asthma continues to increase. There are now an estimated three million asthma sufferers in the UK. The resources required, in terms of manpower and funding to manage these patients, continues to rise in primary care as more prophylactic therapy is, justifiably, prescribed.

Organised asthma care in the community, usually in the form of asthma clinics, became officially recognised in 1990. Since then, the emphasis of care has shifted from secondary to primary care. Many practice nurses, district nurses, health visitors and school nurses are now playing a very important role in the delivery of preventive asthma care. They have become the major providers of asthma education for patients and their families. General practitioners continue to see many asthma patients, particularly for the diagnosis and acute management of the condition.

1

The hospital team, from the chest physician through to the respiratory nurse, physiotherapist and lung function technician all have an important role to play. It is vital that both the hospital and primary care teams deliver a consistent approach embracing current modern asthma management.

"**Asthma: Ask the Experts**" provides answers to highly topical questions which will be of value to all health professionals regardless of where they work. Topics include up-to-date information on asthma and allergy, ranging from the size of the problem to the importance of the environment and the prospects for primary prevention. The chapter on paediatric asthma includes problems of diagnosis and treatment of the under twos and the risk versus benefits of inhaled corticosteroids in children. Adult asthma is comprehensively covered and looks at differential diagnoses, brittle asthma and occupational asthma. Also included here is information about recently introduced asthma drugs and an assessment of new inhaler delivery systems. A further chapter is devoted to patient education and compliance issues, the role of self-management and the value of quality of life questionnaires. The final chapter answers a miscellany of questions and includes answers on the cost implications of intensive primary care management, the importance of audit and outcome measures and the value of guidelines. Shared care and the role of the asthma nurse in the community and the hospital are also addressed.

"**Asthma: Ask the Experts**" has been written to celebrate the 10th Anniversary of the founding of the National Asthma Training Centre in 1987. The Centre, which has charitable status, has, to date, trained over 15,000 health professionals nationwide as well as introducing training programmes overseas.

The large National Asthma Training Centre training network, of 300 Trainers and Instructors, has allowed us to develop and "spread the message". This would not, however, have been possible without the support and encouragement of eminent members of the medical profession. All the authors of "**Asthma: Ask the Experts**" have, in one way or another, contributed to the development of the National Asthma Training Centre.

The 10th Anniversary seemed an excellent opportunity to bring together these experts, all of whom have so much to offer, be they a professor, chest physician, GP or specialist nurse. I am extremely grateful to all the contributors who answered their question with such willingness (and only a very little nagging on my behalf) without any form of remuneration. They are all true experts. They are people who have a special skill and knowledge and are prepared to share it with others. My heartfelt thanks to them all.

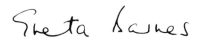

Chapter 1

The Background: Prevalence, mechanisms and triggers

Peter Burney

Professor Peter G.J. Burney, MA, MD, MRCP, FFPHM, is Professor of Public Health Medicine and Chairman of the Division of Public Health Services at the United Medical and Dental Schools of Guy's and St Thomas's Hospitals, London.

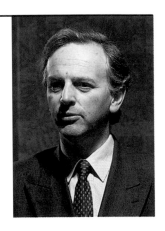

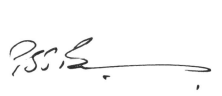

1
Is asthma really on the increase?

The main evidence for an increase in asthma over the last quarter of a century comes from approximately 50 studies from around the world that have measured the prevalence of the disease on more than one occasion in the same population. Some of these surveys have asked people about whether they have asthma, and others have asked about symptoms, such as wheeze, that are associated with asthma. Almost without exception, these studies show an increase over time.

This evidence alone, however, is less than conclusive because the changes could reflect the way that people respond to and report disease rather than any real changes in the prevalence of underlying disease. In the 1980s, doctors were encouraged to diagnose and treat asthma more readily than they had been before, and it is argued that this may have increased the number of people with asthma who recognised that they had the condition without any change in the real number of people with asthma. This view draws some support from the fact that the prevalence of reported asthma has increased in some studies faster than the prevalence of symptoms such as wheeze.

Circumstantial evidence that the increase in asthma is real comes from the observation that the other atopic conditions, such as hay fever and eczema, also appear to be increasing, though there is generally less evidence on these than on asthma, and that the treatment rates for asthma both in hospital and   5 in general practice have increased over the same time. Such evidence, however, has the same weaknesses as the original evidence. It is possible that the other atopic conditions are recognised more because they are treated more, and the increase in treatment rates may be more to do with doctors' and patients' behaviour than with any real increase in disease.

More objective evidence for an increase in asthma could come from physiological measures made over time, but there are far fewer such studies and their results are not always consistent. Two studies of school children, one in Switzerland and one in Japan, have shown that there have been increases over time in the proportion of children who produce specific immunoglobulin E (IgE) antibodies to common allergens, and an increase in atopic diseases including asthma would be expected to follow from this. Another study of Australian school children did not show an increase in skin sensitivity over time, though it did show an increase in bronchial reactivity (a common feature of asthma). This increase in bronchial reactivity has also been shown to have increased in a survey of school children in south Wales. However, a study of adults in Australia failed to show such an increase, even though there had been an increase in symptoms.

The balance of evidence is in favour of a real increase in asthma over the last quarter of a century. The plausibility of this is greatly increased by the emerging evidence for very great variations in disease between places. Such evidence is much easier to document than the historical record.

Julian Hopkin

Dr Julian M. Hopkin, MD, MA, MSc, FRCP, is Senior Clinical Lecturer at the University of Oxford.

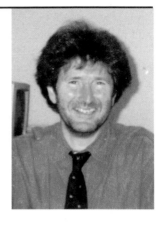

2
Is asthma all in the genes?

The short answer to this question is: "Certainly not". Asthma is a syndrome which has many causes. In some instances these are entirely environmental, as is the case, for example, with heavy isocyanate exposure in industry. For most people with asthma, those between the ages of 5 and 30, the principal cause is atopy, or allergy to common inhaled dusts. The underlying causes of atopy are mixed and there is undoubtedly interaction between a number of genetic effects and various environmental influences.

Asthma is on the increase in Western countries. It is also the case that migrants to Western countries acquire higher rates of asthma. Both these observations point strongly to an important environmental change, or factor (S), in developed countries in recent decades. The nature of this change/factor is obscure. Personally, I wonder whether exposure to certain infections, either as the result of improved living standards or immunisation schedules, might be the key.

What then of the genetics? It is clear from twin studies that genetic factors are also important in determining risk of atopy underlying asthma. A number of molecular genetic studies on atopy and asthma are now in progress and it is clear that variants/mutants in a number of genes, and affecting different proteins/functions in the immune system, participate.

After a controversial start, we now know that a gene on chromosome 11 is important and that its variants probably act by affecting the immu-　7 noglobulin E (IgE) receptor on mast cells in the bronchus. Other genetic effects have been provisionally located to chromosomes 5, 13 and 16, but it is unclear which genes are involved and how their variants affect the immune system to promote atopy. No "asthma gene", as such, has been identified yet. It is interesting that variants of another gene, controlling production of mast cell chymase which causes skin inflammation, is strongly related to the risk of the allergic skin disease, eczema. A good deal of work remains to be done in finally identifying the major genetic effects, and this is an important area of future research.

The prevention of asthma, on the scale that we now know it, depends on our achieving an understanding of both the genetic and the environmental factors that promote the disease.

Kevin Jones

Dr Kevin Jones, MA, DM, MRCGP, is Senior Lecturer in Primary Health Care at the University of Newcastle-upon-Tyne.

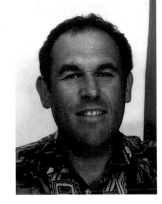

3
Does ethnicity influence the prevalence and severity of asthma?

Ethnic origin plays a major part in the epidemiology of many important chronic diseases and so it is pertinent to consider what effect, if any, it has in asthma. Published literature reveals three separate sets of studies– from the United Kingdom, New Zealand and the United States—which may help to illuminate this point.

In the United Kingdom, work in Blackburn published in 1987 examined the clinical impression that asthma admissions among ethnic Asian adults were more frequent than expected, concluding that there was a raised rate in this group which was not due to increased readmissions. This work was revisited in 1991–92 when the same difference was observed. The authors concluded that either asthma prevalence was higher in this group or that cultural factors might explain the observed difference—a very broad conclusion indeed!

Research in Southampton in 1989–90 sought to compare the prevalence of asthma in Asian and European children. No differences in prevalence were found between the two groups. The researchers suggested that the apparent differences in prevalence reported from primary care might result from either more severe or less adequately treated asthma among Asians or from a lower threshold for seeking medical attention in this group. The latter point is not clearly supported by published evidence, but there are data from London in 1990–91 which indicate that the risk of under-

9

diagnosis and under-treatment was higher at that time in children from ethnic minority groups. Intriguingly, there is a suggestion that it might be more common for foods—especially ice, fizzy drinks, fried food and nuts (particularly betel nuts)—to act as a trigger to asthma in Asians. Whether this means that Asians eat more of such foods or are any more likely to react to them is unclear.

Studies from New Zealand in the 1980s reported that the asthma mortality rate in that country was much higher in Pacific Islanders or Polynesians (9.4 per 100,000) and Maoris (18.9) than in Caucasians (3.4). Paediatric admission and readmission rates (as well as length of stay) followed the same pattern. Particularly in children, it was concluded that such differences could not be explained by genetic or socio-economic factors but related more to patterns of medical management such as: inadequate long-term medical care, under-estimation of severity by family and doctors, failure to call for help when needed and inadequate responses from medical services. Major ethnic differences in asthma drug management, both in the community and at the time of hospital discharge, were also noted. Research published in 1994 still revealed that asthma symptoms were more commonly found among Maoris compared with other groups.

Research on asthma admission and mortality rates in New York City reveals that these events occur between three and five and a half times more commonly among Black and Hispanic populations than among White. No explanations were offered for these differences.

The conclusions of these various pieces of research indicate that a simple, clear answer to the question posed cannot be given at this time—as ever, more research is needed. Few, if any, studies in the UK have truly addressed the issue of ethnic differences in asthma incidence and prevalence on a population basis. However, it appears likely that the major determinant of differences in the apparent prevalence and severity of asthma between ethnic groups lies more in the cultural experience, attitudes and expectations of such groups and their health carers than in the genes they each carry. It is therefore a challenge to all those caring for people with asthma that a high standard of management, education and treatment should be given to all, irrespective of their ethnic origin.

Martin Church

Professor Martin K. Church, MPharm, PhD, DSc,
is Professor of Experimental
Immunopharmacology at the University of
Southampton.

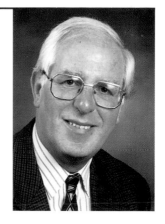

4
Why do people have allergic responses?

In the civilised world, we usually think of allergy as just "bad news". But, really, would evolution have facilitated the development of such a response unless it had some use? Of course not!

To begin to understand the positive aspects of the allergic response, we need to move our thoughts to the developing countries where parasitic infestation is rife. The problem with parasites is that they are massive in comparison with the viruses and bacteria which the neutrophils and macrophages of the immune system usually have to deal with. The evolutionary solution to this problem is what we regard as the allergic response, i.e., a whole tissue response which makes the local environment as hostile as possible to the invading parasite.

In the intestine, smooth contraction (seen as diarrhoea), increased blood flow to recruit inflammatory leucocytes, increased mucus production and the sacrifice of epithelial cells are all stimulated in an attempt to prevent a parasite from gaining entry into the body. Exactly the same events are seen in intestinal allergy. Bearing in mind that the lung is derived from the gut during embryo development, is it surprising that an essentially similar response occurs in the airways? In the lung, the response manifests as asthma. In the eye and nasal mucosae, which do not have underlying smooth muscle, increased blood flow and itching (a further physical defence system) predominate.

11

Based on these observations, we can define allergy as a condition in which sensitive individuals recognise harmless proteins, usually enzymes, such as house dust mite or pollen allergens, as though they were parasite antigens and then respond to them with immunoglobulin E (IgE) synthesis. Following a second exposure to these proteins, which the body wrongly believes to be a parasite trying to enter the body, the sensitised individual's immune system responds in a totally inappropriate fashion.

So, a response which, when mounted against its natural target, namely a living parasite, helps to reduce reinfestation in millions of people in the developing world, gives rise, when mounted against an inappropriate target, to a debilitating and often chronic allergic response. Perhaps the situation is best summarised by adapting a traditional saying to read: "one man's immune defence is another man's allergy".

Stephen Holgate

Professor Stephen Holgate, MD, DSc, FRCP, is
MRC Clinical Professor of Immunopharmacology
at the University of Southampton.

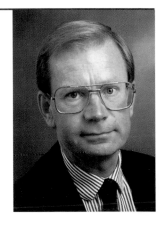

Stephen T. Holgate

5
What are the cellular mechanisms of asthma?

Asthma is a disorder in which the airways which carry air in and out of the
lungs contract too easily and too much. This may occur spontaneously or,
commonly, in response to a variety of external factors, including exposure
to allergens, viral infections, exercise, cold air, fog and irritant fumes, as well
as internal factors, including laughing, at night time and with stress.

It is important to ask why asthmatic airways behave in this way.
Asthma was at one time thought of as a spasmodic disease. However,
while symptoms of asthma are frequently spasmodic, the underlying
mechanisms are commonly persistent, although varying in severity. Our
understanding of asthma has greatly increased by recognising that underlying the symptoms is a special type of inflammation of the airways, involving special cells (called mast cells and eosinophils). In asthma, but not in
normal people, these cells secrete a range of chemical substances (called
mediators) that cause the airways to narrow either alone or when aggra-
vated by an external agent.

The most common form of asthma occurs in association with allergy to
common environmental agents—for example, house dust mites, pets and
fungi—most frequently encountered in the home. Repeated exposure to
these agents in those who inherit certain genes for allergy and asthma, leads
to the formation of a special protein called immunoglobulin E (IgE). IgE is
an antibody, part of a group of proteins whose job it is to protect us against   13

foreign organisms. However, in asthma this IgE is in part responsible for triggering the release of mediators from the mast cells and eosinophils.

Another important cell in asthma is the T lymphocyte—a small round cell forming another part of our immune system. In asthma, but not in normal people, these cells in the airways become stimulated by common allergens, such as those from house dust mites, to secrete a range of small proteins (called cytokines). The purpose of these proteins is to bring in fresh mast cells and eosinophils and create a comfortable environment for them to survive. They also lead to increased production of the antibody, IgE. The net result of this inflammation is to create the spasmodic symptoms of asthma. Over time, the inflammation also changes the structure of the airways, causing the disease to be chronic and less easily treated.

Anti-asthma drugs, such as cromoglycate and the inhaled corticosteroids, budesonide, beclomethasone and fluticasone, control the inflammation and, therefore, the symptoms of asthma. However, they must be taken regularly. For reasons explained above, it is also important that asthma is recognised early and that appropriate anti-inflammatory treatment is given to prevent progression of the disorder and to enable people to lead normal lives.

John Warner

Professor John O. Warner, MD, FRCP, DCH, is
Professor of Child Health at the University of
Southampton.

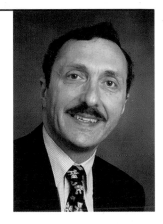

6
Does sensitisation occur in utero?

The simple answer is "Yes". It has been known for many years that a raised
level of allergy antibody immunoglobulin E (IgE) in the cord blood is a
highly specific, though not particularly sensitive, predictor of subsequent
allergic disease. In other words, virtually all newborn infants with a raised
IgE at birth develop allergic problems within one to three years but most
children with allergy have had a normal IgE level at birth. Occasionally,
allergy antibodies to cows' milk have been detected in the cord blood and
these data suggest that at least occasionally sensitisation does occur in utero.

More recently, my own group has demonstrated that much more frequently than finding a raised IgE in the cord blood we find that the white
blood cells known as lymphocytes are sensitised to a range of allergens—not
only food but also inhalants—in newborns who subsequently develop
allergic disease. This in utero sensitisation is common and may occur in
virtually all fetuses. How this relates to the subsequent development of
asthma and allergy remains to be established. We have, however, shown that
only some newborns' lymphocytes have an allergic characteristic of response
generating messenger substances which promote the development of IgE.
We have also shown that this sensitisation process is influenced by the
concentration of exposure of the mother both to inhalant and ingestant
allergens. The timing of sensitisation is from 22 weeks' gestation and
onwards, which is rather earlier than has hitherto been thought to be the case. 15

The implications of these observations are enormous. They raise the issue of whether strategies for preventing sensitisation by maternal avoidance during pregnancy will be necessary. However, recommendations should not be made until further more detailed research studies have been completed. There are dangers to recommending dietary avoidance during pregnancy, particularly as this might compromise nutrition not only of the mother but also of the growing fetus. Indeed there is some evidence that such compromise might even increase the risk of allergy. For the present, however, the most important implication is that a significant number of newborns who will go on to develop allergic problems will be identifiable at birth. Such identification will provide an opportunity to initiate avoidance and other therapy at an early stage which might have the possibility of altering the long-term natural history of the problem. Some fetuses and infants who develop sensitisation subsequently do not develop disease.

David Strachan

Dr David Strachan, MD, MSc, MRCGP, FFPHM,
is Reader in Epidemiology at St George's
Hospital Medical School, London.

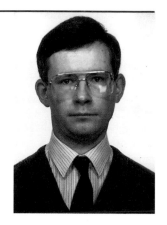

David Strachan

7
Does the indoor environment affect asthma?

The indoor air in homes, workplaces and other buildings may contain small quantities of irritant gases, airborne particles and allergens, any of which may affect the occurrence of asthma. We need to consider two rather different questions.

First, we need to look at whether the indoor environment triggers attacks, or makes asthma symptoms worse, among people who already have the disease. There is ample anecdotal evidence that asthmatics experience worsening of symptoms on exposure to indoor allergens to which they are already allergic, such as the neighbour's cat. This is supported by scientific experiments on volunteers exposed to small quantities of allergens such as house dust mite. There is less consistent experimental evidence of adverse effects from exposure to indoor particles and irritants. One irritant gas to which asthmatics are known to be especially sensitive, sulphur dioxide, is present only at very low concentrations in most homes in Great Britain.

A few experimental studies have been carried out to see if modifications to the indoor environment improve asthma symptoms. These have mainly focused on reducing allergen exposure, particularly from house dust mites. Symptoms usually improve when mite-allergic asthmatics live for several months in environments totally free of mites, but it has proved extremely difficult to reduce mite allergen exposure substantially by simple and   17 acceptable modifications to most British homes. However, many of the studies so far have been too small to demonstrate a subtle but possibly beneficial effect and more research is required in this area.

Second, we need to consider whether the indoor environment causes healthy people to develop asthma. The evidence here is much less convincing. Several studies, particularly those of young children, have shown that wheezing is more common in homes where parents smoke (an avoidable source of airborne particles and irritants). It is not clear whether this reflects indoor air pollution or the effects on the developing lungs of mothers smoking during pregnancy. A few studies have found more asthma in homes where gas is used for cooking (a source of the irritant gas nitrogen dioxide). However, other research shows no such relationship and the link between gas cooking and asthma is far from proven.

There has been speculation for many years that the amount of allergen exposure, particularly early in life, may affect the risk of developing asthma. Specific allergies, for instance to house dust or pets, are indeed related to the amount of exposure to the relevant indoor allergen. These allergies are, in turn, more closely related to asthma than, for instance, pollen allergy. However, the evidence linking allergen exposure directly to the risk of developing asthma is weak and inconsistent. This may be because we do not yet have accurate enough measurements of exposure, for instance to airborne allergen (rather than allergens in carpet dust), or of allergens encountered at some critical period early in life. It may also be that families with allergy take measures to avoid indoor allergens (by choice of bedding or by avoiding pets) and this tends to obscure a true relationship between allergen exposure and asthma risk.

Ross Anderson

Professor H. Ross Anderson, MD, MSc, FFPHM,
is Professor of Epidemiology and Public Health at
St George's Hospital Medical School, London.

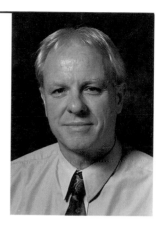

8
Does the outdoor environment affect asthma?

There are three main outdoor environmental factors that may affect
asthma—weather, outdoor pollution and aero-allergens (pollens and
mould spores).

Asthma shows a strong seasonal cycle. The most obvious feature is an
increase in the autumn, and suggested explanations include sudden drops
in temperature, autumn mould spores, increased growth of house dust
mites (due to increased humidity) or epidemics of respiratory infections
associated with the return of children to school. We do not know the
relative importance of these at either a public health or individual level.
Thunderstorms are sometimes associated with asthma epidemics, probably through some kind of allergic reaction to pollens which have been
modified by damp air.

Pollens are a potent cause of hay fever but are less important in asthma
because they are too large to be inhaled deep into the airways. Nevertheless,
there is a small rise in asthma during the pollen season. The main sources of
aero-allergens are various moulds, especially those which tend to discharge
spores in the autumn; we do not know much about their role.

There is current concern about the role of air pollution as a cause of
asthma as well as an aggravating factor in persons who already have asthma.
The possibility that the increase in asthma is due to increased exposure to
motor vehicle emissions has been raised. The important ambient pollutants   19

which could be responsible are nitrogen dioxide, small particles, sulphur dioxide and ozone (a secondary pollutant formed downwind from pollution sources when there is sunny weather). There is good evidence that some individuals with asthma may be made worse by inhaling motor vehicle fumes and other forms of pollution. Evidence from the United Kingdom and other countries shows that hospital attendances for asthma are a little higher on high pollution days and that this may be due to the irritating effects of a range of pollutants. Recent studies have also found a higher prevalence of asthma near busy roads, especially those carrying heavy vehicles. This may point to an effect of air pollution and is being investigated further. Nevertheless, it is generally agreed that, at a public health level, air pollution plays a relatively small role in the aggravation of asthma; other factors such as those responsible for seasonal variations (above), infections and allergens are much more important.

While outdoor air pollution plays a role in the provocation or aggravation of existing asthma, there is very little evidence that it is responsible for the initiation of the asthmatic disease itself. The rise in asthma which has occurred in the United Kingdom and other parts of the world is not thought to be explained by changes in air pollution. This view is supported by the observation that the increase in asthma has accompanied an overall reduction in air pollution and that the prevalence of asthma is similar in rural and urban areas. In addition, asthma has increased to a marked degree in some countries such as New Zealand where air pollution levels are low.

Jill Warner

Dr Jill Warner, PhD, is Senior Lecturer in Allergy and Immunology in the Department of Child Health at the University of Southampton.

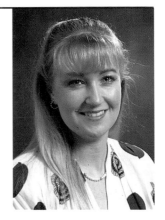

9
What are the prospects for primary prevention of asthma?

The highly allergic nature of paediatric asthma has led to much interest in attempting to reproduce, in a normal domestic environment, the extremely successful action of sending asthmatic children to special schools at high altitude where allergens and adjuvants of allergic disease are minimal. There is now great interest in whether this effective allergen avoidance in early life can prevent asthma from developing at all.

Avoidance of exposure to high concentrations of allergens in the first year of life reduces the risk of allergic sensitisation, whilst high allergen exposure at this time is associated with earlier onset of wheeze in asthmatic individuals. One study from the Isle of Wight has shown a reduction in the development of allergy in a group of high-risk children where avoidance of food (cow's milk, egg, fish and nuts) and house dust mite allergens was implemented at birth, compared with high-risk children where no environmental manipulation was performed.

We have shown that peripheral blood mononuclear cell (PBMC) proliferative responses and cytokine profiles to specific allergens are already altered at birth in babies who subsequently develop allergic disease compared to those with no disease. We have also shown that positive PBMC proliferative responses to specific allergens can be detected from 22 weeks' gestation, and that these responses were higher in babies whose mothers were exposed to increased allergen concentrations after 22 weeks of 21 pregnancy. Antenatal factors, including maternal and thereby fetal exposure to allergens and tobacco smoke, are therefore critical for the development of asthma in genetically predisposed individuals.

Cell-mediated immunity is detrimental to the pregnant state and there is a damping of this response in the maternal system with a concurrent move towards humeral immunity. This is mediated by a switch in the T helper cell population of the feto-placental unit to produce Th2 cytokines (Interleukins 4, 5 and 10) which inhibit maternal Th1 chtokine production (IL-2, Interferon gamma (IFN-γ) and Tumour necrosis factor beta (TNF-β). Therefore, by producing Th2-like cytokines the feto-placental unit blocks the maternal cell-mediated responses which would compromise fetal survival. However, the production of Th2 cytokines promotes allergy, whilst Th1 cytokines suppress allergy.

Preliminary results show that PBMCs from most fetuses spontaneously release IFN-γ during the 2nd and 3rd trimesters of pregnancy, but that there are some which do not release this Th1 cytokine. We hypothesise that the role of non-specific fetal PBMC IFN-γ production is to counteract the effects of allergy-promoting cytokines produced by the placenta and/or mother. A mechanism such as this would be essential to prevent an allergic (Th-2) phenotype in all newborns. Failure of this mechanism may underlie the development of atopy.

Our current research strategy is therefore to investigate the hypothesis that environmental modification through pregnancy and early infancy will prevent the development of allergy and asthma. We have just commenced enrolment of a cohort of families with allergic asthma into our Child Health Asthma Prevention Study (CHAPS). For this study, an intensive allergen avoidance programme is being instituted from 18 weeks of pregnancy and continued through the child's first year of life in a controlled trial to establish whether avoidance will reduce the prevalence of asthma. The already existing level of knowledge about the timing of the development of the altered immune responses associated with the development of allergy and asthma would suggest that, if effective maternal and infant avoidance of house dust mite and pet allergens can be achieved, there are very good prospects for primary prevention of asthma.

Jane Hubbard

Jane Hubbard, SRN, NATC Dip in Asthma Care, is
a Practice Nurse in Kingston-upon-Thames and a
National Asthma Training Centre Regional
Trainer.

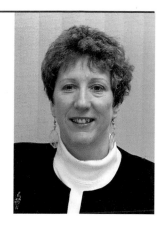

Jane Hubbard

10
**What advice should be given to a couple contemplating pregnancy who
have a strong family history of asthma?**

Prospective parents with a strong family history of asthma should be told
that their children do have an increased chance of developing asthma, but
that it is possible to take various measures to reduce this chance.

Asthma is not inherited as a single gene disorder, unlike, for example,
cystic fibrosis. At present, pending further research, a positive family history
of atopic (IgE mediated) disease is the best predictor of risk. Children born
to a couple with a strong family history of atopy have a 30–60% chance of
developing an allergic disorder. The chance is increased if both parents are
affected. Boys are more at risk than girls. Some but not all studies suggest
that maternal history is more important than paternal. This stronger
maternal influence could be genetic but could also be due to environmental
effects sensitising the baby in utero.

There is increasing evidence that the timing, nature and level of allergen
exposure in early life may be crucial to the later development of asthma.
Babies born to atopic mothers exhibit delayed maturation of their immune
system in the first weeks of life. Exposure to allergens, such as house dust
mite, animals or pollens, at this time may cause the immune system to
switch to an "allergic" drive instead of developing tolerance to what are, in
reality, harmless substances. Other factors, such as prematurity and low
birth weight, may also be involved.

The most important advice for future parents with a strong history of asthma is not to smoke. Maternal smoking in pregnancy is associated with abnormal lung function in the infant at birth and with altered immune responses which result in increased levels of IgE. It is possible that some infants who are genetically programmed to be at low risk of developing allergy may be converted to high risk by this effect on IgE synthesis. Smoking should also be avoided after the child is born. Post natal exposure to tobacco smoke is causally linked with an increased frequency and severity of asthma symptoms in asthmatic children.

The relationship between infant feeding practices and atopic disease has been extensively researched but results remain inconclusive. However, there is some evidence that the development of asthma in a child may be delayed if the mother avoids certain foods while breast-feeding and also postpones introducing her infant to those foods on weaning. Foods that might be best avoided at these times include dairy products, eggs, wheat, fish, citrus fruits and nuts.

Research is also currently in progress into the effect of controlling allergens, particularly house dust mite and cat, both during pregnancy and post natally. Like the dietary measures already described, measures taken against airborne allergens may have a role in delaying the onset of asthma in infants. This is especially important in view of the difficulties involved in managing asthma in very young children.

The role of pollutants and infections in the development of asthma remains controversial and inconclusive at present. It is possible that respiratory infections in early life may protect against allergic disease by preventing the immune system from switching to allergic responses. However, it is certainly the case that respiratory infections remain important triggers of asthma attacks in asthmatic children.

Thomas Platts-Mills

Professor Thomas Platts-Mills, MD, PhD, is Head
of the Division of Asthma, Allergy and
Immunology and Director of the UVA Asthma
and Allergic Disease Center, Charlottesville,
Virginia, USA.

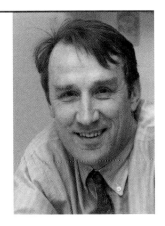

11
What is the role of indoor allergens in asthma?

In most Western countries children and adults spend at least 90% of their
time indoors. Thus the bulk of the immunologically foreign protein that
they inhale is derived from indoor sources such as dust mites, cats, dogs and,
in some areas, cockroaches. The argument that these proteins cause asthma,
or contribute to symptoms of asthma, is based on several types of evidence.
First, there is a very strong association between sensitisation to indoor
allergens and asthma. Sensitisation can be assessed by skin testing or by
radioallergosorbent testing (RAST) of immunoglobulin E (IgE) antibodies.
Second, bronchial provocation with allergen can produce the symptoms of
asthma, decreased lung function and eosinophilic inflammation typical of
asthma. Third, reducing exposure to allergens can improve symptoms. This
latter conclusion is based both on moving patients to sanatoria or allergen
free units in hospital, and also to controlled trials of dust mite allergen
avoidance in the patients' houses. Taken together, the evidence provides
very convincing evidence that exposure to indoor allergens is an important
cause of asthma and that allergen avoidance should be regarded as a first line
anti-inflammatory treatment for asthma.

There are of course some problems with this theory; in most cases the
patients are not aware that they are allergic to house dust allergens and do
not recognise the role that these allergens play in their disease. This is
particularly true for dust mite but also for cockroach allergic individuals.   25

The explanation for this appears to be that patients become relatively insensitive to nasal symptoms with daily exposure, and, more important, that inhalation of a relatively small number of dust mite faecal particles (20 to 200) would not be expected to produce detectable decreases in pulmonary function but could nonetheless produce multiple foci of inflammation in the lungs. Thus the true role of indoor allergens in asthma may be as a chronic contribution to inflammation of the lungs and the associated bronchial reactivity. Another problem is that avoidance protocols are difficult to carry out, and, even for dust mite, may not be completely effective. Despite these problems, the logical conclusion is that inhaling allergens in houses contributes to sensitisation and asthma symptoms. Thus if patients are sensitised to allergens which are prevalent in an area, or are known to be exposed to them, then avoidance measures should be recommended. Given that the increases in asthma are in perennial disease and that the bulk of the patients are allergic to indoor allergens, it is very likely that increased exposure to these proteins has contributed to the epidemic.

Ashley Woodcock

Dr Ashley Woodcock, BSc, MB ChB, MD, FRCP, is Consultant Respiratory Physician at the North West Lung Centre, Wythenshaw Hospital, Manchester.

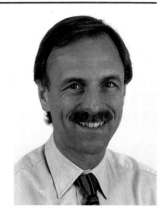

12
Is it possible to eliminate allergens from the home environment?

Minimising the impact of identified environmental risk factors, such as house dust mite, cat and dog allergens, is a critical first management step in reducing the severity of asthma. Although environmental control is difficult, it must become an integral part of the overall management of sensitised asthmatic patients.

Effective reductions in allergen exposure in sensitised asthmatics are undoubtedly associated with improvement in symptoms. For example, mite sensitive children taken to altitude in Switzerland show a progressive improvement in bronchial irritability and reductions in symptoms and medication. The challenge is to create low allergen exposure in patients' homes in the UK and elsewhere.

Integrated strategies for reducing allergen exposure should be flexible enough to be suited to individual needs and at the same time must also be affordable. Allergens from mites and pets have dramatically different aerodynamic characteristics. Dust mite allergens can only be detected after vigorous disturbance whilst airborne dog and cat allergens are readily measured in homes without any artificial disturbance. A critically important proportion of pet allergens are of small particle size which can be inhaled directly. These characteristics underline the differences in the clinical response so that patients who are allergic to house dust mite are usually unaware of the relationship whereas patients sensitive to pets   27 become immediately aware, even on entering a room where a cat has previously been.

For house dust mite avoidance, the single most effective measure is to cover mattresses, pillows and duvets with covers that are impermeable to mite allergens. These covers were initially made of plastic and were uncomfortable to sleep on, but water vapour permeable fabrics have since been developed which are both impermeable to mite allergen and comfortable to sleep on. Allergen levels are dramatically reduced after the introduction of such covers. All exposed bedding should be washed at high temperature to kill mites and remove allergen. Ideally, carpets should be replaced with wood/vinyl flooring and curtains should be washed. In this way, dust mite exposure in bed at night can be virtually abolished.

Intensive vacuum cleaning with high filtration cleaners reduces the size of the dust mite allergen reservoir but no benefit has been established in a clinical trial. Killing mites with chemicals is feasible in the laboratory but is not clinically effective. Air filters and ionisers are of no clinical benefit. Large numbers of mite allergen control products are currently available but claims for their clinical efficacy are often exaggerated and inadequately tested. An integrated approach to dust mite avoidance (i.e., bed covers, dust removal and removal of carpets) is undoubtedly the best.

The avoidance of pet allergens is more problematic. Pet allergens are present in huge concentrations in houses with cats or dogs but they also transfer on clothing so that levels are detectable in homes without pets and even in hospital outpatient areas. The best way to reduce exposure to animal allergens is to get rid of the family pet but this is often not practicable. Even after permanent removal of a cat from a home it can take many months before the reservoir allergen levels return to normal. So, if patients do decide to get rid of their pet, they should be told not to expect to get better immediately.

For patients who choose to keep their pets, it is important that they should keep their animals out of the bedroom and living room. Measures such as the use of air filters, regular thorough vacuum cleaning of carpets and weekly washing of animals all reduce allergen levels, although the size of the clinical benefit has not been established.

It is apparent that allergen levels can be reduced sufficiently to prevent sensitised patients from reacting within their own home environment. The critical issue at this point is whether allergen levels can be reduced sufficiently to prevent initial sensitisation in early life.

Samantha Walker

Samantha Walker, RGN, NATC Dip in Asthma
Care, is Clinical Research Sister at the Royal
Brompton Hospital, London.

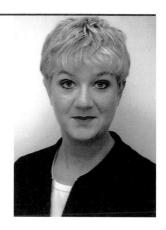

13
What practical measures can be taken to reduce allergen levels in the home?

Ideally the best way of reducing exposure to indoor allergens would be to remove those allergens completely from the patient's environment. Currently it is impossible to eradicate allergens from inside the home but various measures for avoiding house dust mite and animal allergens can be helpful.

Before embarking on avoidance measures, it is important to check that the patient's history suggests clinical sensitivity to the allergen, as the measures given here may not be appropriate for all patients. Suggestions for avoiding house dust mites are:

- Have a bed with a plain wooden base, not a divan.
- Use synthetic duvets and pillows.
- Replace the mattress if it is an old one.
- Cover mattresses, pillows and duvets with dust proof covers (ideally these should have been shown to be effective in clinical trials). Mattress covers should fully enclose the mattress and should be zippable.
- Use bedding that allows a hot wash (over 60°C) on a weekly basis.
- Remove carpets and either have bare floorboards or cover with vinyl flooring. Have small washable rugs if desired.
- Do not allow animals into the bedroom (mite counts have been shown to be higher in areas frequented by cats and dogs).

29

- Have thin, washable curtains or roller blinds.
- Reduce soft toys to a minimum and keep them in a closed box when not being played with. Machine-wash soft toys regularly at a high temperature (over 60°C) or place them in the deep freeze overnight. These measures will kill the mites. The toys should then be vacuumed to remove the dead mites.
- Use a vacuum cleaner with a filter that retains allergen and stops it being distributed around the room. (The British Allergy Foundation have approved some of these.)
- Air filters, ionisers and various acaricides (chemicals which kill mites) may be of value although there is no proof of their effectiveness at the present time.

Suggestions for avoiding animal allergens (which remain airborne for many hours and may provoke symptoms even in the absence of the animal) are:

- Avoid having furry animals in the house, especially in the bedroom.
- Do not buy or replace pets in the future.
- Continue to clean the home vigorously for a prolonged period (possibly for up to six months) after removal of a pet.
- Where removal of a pet is not possible, keep the animal outside or in an area which has washable flooring. This will minimise the accumulation of allergen particles.
- Vacuum the house regularly using a vacuum cleaner approved by the British Allergy Foundation. The filters in these models stop animal allergen being blown around.
- Have bare wooden floors or vinyl floor coverings. Carpets and underfelt act as a reservoir for allergen, and so removing carpeting will help reduce allergen levels.
- Ensure that animals' bedding is changed or washed regularly.
- Wash cats once a week. Recent studies have suggested that this, when combined with other cleaning measures, may effectively reduce cat allergen levels in the home.

Anthony Frew

Dr Anthony J. Frew, MA, MD, MRCP, is Senior Lecturer in Medicine at the University of Southampton and Honorary Consultant Physician at the Allergy and Asthma Clinic, Southampton General Hospital.

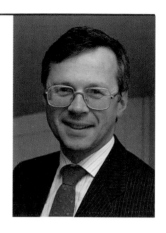

14
How are relevant allergens identified?

Allergens are foreign molecules which are recognised by immunoglobulin E (IgE) antibodies and can trigger allergic reactions. The term "antigen" is used for any molecule which is recognised by T lymphocytes or any type of antibody. Allergens are thus a restricted subset of antigens. Strictly speaking, an allergen is a single component of a protein extract, although in common parlance people often use the term allergen to describe pollens, mites, moulds, animal dander, etc. When a substance is thought to cause allergy, an extract can be prepared from a suitable source material and then used for skin testing. If the extract is properly prepared and standardised, a positive skin reaction will include the presence of IgE antibodies and may implicate that allergenic material as the cause of that patient's allergy. It is important to make sure there is no irritant material in the extract which could cause false-positive reactions.

To identify individual allergens within a mixture, the protein extract is run on a gel to separate the different components. Extracts from house dust mite, pollen, cat dander, etc., may contain between 15 and 20 different proteins, most of which are not allergenic. To identify which of the proteins are relevant allergens, we take serum from several patients and layer this on top of the gel containing the protein extract. After washing the gel we can then look to see where IgE antibodies have bound in the gel. Having identified the proteins which bind IgE (the allergens) the next phase is to 31 assess the portion of allergic subjects who react against individual proteins. To do this we take sera from a large panel of patients who have positive skin test reactions to the allergen extract, and then we look to see which of the protein bands bind to the individual sera. Proteins which are recognised by more than half of the allergic patients are termed major allergens. Those proteins recognised by a minority of patient sera are termed minor allergens. Proteins which are not recognised by any of the allergic sera are regarded as non-allergenic. Once a major allergen has been identified it is possible to develop assays to determine how much of that major allergen is present in the environment. This is particularly useful for house dust mite and cat dander.

For skin testing in clinical practice we need an extract that contains all the major allergens and most of the minor allergens in the proportions that they occur naturally. This should make it possible to detect all patients who react to the allergenic components of an extract and also give some indication of the degree of sensitivity.

Susan Cross

Susan Cross, RN, SN Cert, NATC Dip in Asthma Care, NP Dip, BSc (Hons), PGCE, is Head of Training at the National Asthma Training Centre.

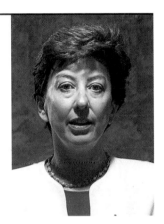

15
What is the value of skin prick testing in general practice and what advice would you give to a practice contemplating introducing it?

Skin prick testing (SPT) has an important role to play in relation to asthma in general practice. Although SPT highlights atopy rather than allergy, it can help confirm the diagnosis. Often the patient will suspect that he or she is "allergic" to a particular trigger, perhaps the pet dog or cat, or a health professional may suspect that persistent symptoms in a patient may be due to sensitivity to a persistent trigger such as house dust mite. Both these scenarios can be confirmed or denied by SPT.

Significant advantages of SPT are that it is less expensive, less time consuming and less invasive than other tests such as radioallergosorbent testing (RAST). Patients with severe and/or chronic disease will often benefit from allergy avoidance advice but this advice can sometimes prove expensive to carry out. By identifying trigger factors in such a visible way, SPT enables patients to see what the problem is and, as a consequence, makes compliance with allergy avoidance more likely.

Before investing in a skin prick testing "kit", a general practice may wish to consider the following points:
- SPT will benefit patients and practice alike if all members of the health care team have an understanding of the benefits and are comfortable that as long as only aero-allergens are used, this is a procedure which, with proper training, can be undertaken safely by a nurse or doctor.

- The technique of SPT is straightforward, but health professionals need a proper level of knowledge to know when to undertake it and how to interpret the results.
- It is advisable to select an independently researched SPT kit with a good record of use in general practice.
- Practice-based SPT is not appropriate for all asthma patients. Referral for specialist assessment is essential in all cases of suspected occupational asthma. Patients with a severe reaction to wasp or bee stings, and those suffering from symptoms of anaphylaxis, should also be referred to an allergy specialist for specific diagnosis, treatment and advice. Testing for food allergies, too, is best performed by a specialist because of the potential risk of anaphylaxis.

Robert Davies

Professor Robert Davies, MA, MD, FRCP, is
Professor of Respiratory Medicine at the London
Chest Hospital.

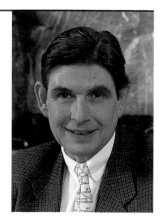

16
How important is air pollution in asthma?

Evidence from a number of epidemiological and laboratory based studies
suggests that there is a clear association between episodes of air pollution
and impaired lung function, respiratory symptoms and hospital Accident
and Emergency Department visits. Although the specific pollutant or pollutants responsible for these effects are not clear, it is thought that the liquid
petroleum and gas-derived air pollutants, namely atmospheric hydro-
carbons, oxides of nitrogen (NO_x), ozone (O_3), sulphur dioxide (SO_2), and
respirable particulate matter (PM_{10}) may be important.

Symptoms of rhinitis and chronic cough and phlegm have been associated with higher personal exposure to NO_2 in adults. Similarly, increased
levels of night time NO_2 have also been associated with decreased mean
morning peak flow in asthmatic children. Continuous monitoring of asthmatics' diary cards and environmental pollution levels have shown that
symptoms, inhaler consumption and peak flow are also significantly wor-
sened, in children and in adults, by increased levels of O_3, with a lag effect of
O_3 exposure maximal between 24 and 48 hours. Similarly, increased levels
of PM_{10} are also related with worsening peak flow, inhaler usage and
respiratory symptoms in asthmatic children and adults, with a lag effect of
one to four days. More recently, large cohort studies have suggested that
there may also be a link between fine particulate pollution and cardio-
pulmonary and lung cancer mortality.

Other studies have suggested that the increased levels of petroleum and gas-generated air pollutants may be linked to increased incidence of allergic disease, particularly in the developed countries. Although early studies from Japan and Germany suggested that there was a significant association between increased vehicle exhaust pollution and increased incidence of rhino-conjunctivitis and hay fever, the findings from these studies have been difficult to interpret due to confounding effects of cigarette smoke, exposure to allergens, meteorological conditions and socio-economic factors. Additionally, these studies have investigated the effects of only the major pollutants individually, without taking into account the potential additive and/or synergistic effects of combinations of pollutants which are more relevant. Recent studies, however, have suggested that the increase in allergic sensitisation is likely to be related to changes in air pollution patterns, lifestyles and living conditions.

Laboratory based studies of asthmatics exposed to O_3, NO_2 and a combination of NO_2 and SO_2 have also indicated that these agents increase the airway responsiveness of these individuals to inhaled allergen. Studies investigating the mechanisms underlying the effects resulting from inhalation of air pollutants have demonstrated that these modulate the activity of immuno-competent cells and increase the synthesis of immunoglobulin E (IgE). Other studies have shown that exposure to pollutants such as O_3 and NO_2 leads to damage and inflammation of the airways. Indeed, in vitro studies have demonstrated that exposure of airway epithelial cells to these pollutants leads to a significant attenuation of ciliary activity, and significant increases in epithelial cell damage, permeability and release of pro-inflammatory mediators.

In conclusion, epidemiological and laboratory based studies provide evidence that exposure to air pollutants generated primarily from burning of liquid petroleum and gas are likely to lead to increased sensitisation of the airways in allergic individuals and to exacerbate the symptoms of their disease. Although the precise mechanisms underlying the effects of these pollutants are not clear, they are likely to potentiate both an easier penetration and access of inhaled allergens to cells of the immune system (as a consequence of decreased ciliary activity and increased epithelial damage and permeability) and also inflammation of the airways (as a consequence of increased synthesis and/or release of pro-inflammatory mediators which influence the differentiation, growth and activity of eosinophils, neutrophils, mast cells, lymphocytes and macrophages).

Rory Shaw

Dr Rory J. Shaw, BSc, MD, MBA, DIC, FRCP, is
Consultant Physician at the Chest & Allergy Clinic
of St Mary's Hospital, London.

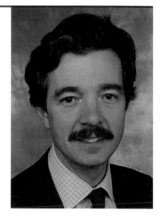

17
Does diet affect asthma?

The question "Does what I eat affect asthma?" is asked frequently by patients. In the majority of cases the presence of asthma and the severity of asthma are unrelated to the type of food in the diet. However, there are a number of situations where there is clear evidence that specific foods or agents in the diet can make asthma worse. These dietary agents can be divided into two main categories: those which cause an acute exacerbation of asthma and those which may contribute to the severity of chronic asthma. The agents which can cause an acute exacerbation of asthma can be further divided into those where the mechanism is immunoglobulin E (IgE) mediated and those where the mechanism is independent of IgE.

In IgE mediated reactions there is an allergen in the food and, where the food item is ingested, an IgE dependent reaction occurs, causing a type I hypersensitivity response. Examples of this include the reactions to peanuts, shellfish, and foods which contain molecules related to latex, such as banana, avocado and kiwi fruit. Also within this category of reaction are IgE mediated type I hypersensitivity responses to allergens in food which cross-react very closely with allergens present in the air, to which the individual is sensitive. An example of this includes the birch pollen allergy syndrome. The principle allergen is birch pollen, which causes hay fever. However, some fruits, such as apples and pears, when eaten raw contain sufficient or cross-reacting allergen for the individual to experience an adverse reaction. 37

The second mechanism by which food causes acute reactions is not mediated via IgE. Histamine is an important mediator of allergic reactions, and certain foods, including certain fish species when they become rotten as well as mature cheese, may contain high concentrations of histamine which can cause an adverse reaction when ingested. Other foods, such as strawberries, can cause the release of histamine from mast cells via a non-IgE dependent mechanism. A further group of agents can cause non-IgE mediated acute reactions to food as a result of a variety of ill-understood mechanisms. These include drugs, such as salicylates (aspirin) and other non-steroidal anti-inflammatory drugs, as well as food additives, such as tartrazine, sulphites, etc.

There has been great debate as to the extent to which chronic asthma, particularly in children, might be exacerbated by exposure to common foods, in particular milk, wheat and eggs. There does appear to be a group of children who experience eczema, asthma and rhinitis in whom avoidance of one of these agents results in clinical benefit, suggesting that the agent might play a role in causing chronic allergic disease in these patients.

Identification of a dietary agent which is exacerbating asthma is difficult. A careful history is essential. In the case of acute asthma, patients usually can identify one or a number of foods which may be exacerbating their condition. The use of diary cards and peak flow meters may be very helpful in adding to the information in the history. Similarly, it may be important to contact the manufacturers of products to identify the nature of additives. Skin tests and radioallergosorbent testing (RAST) may provide supplementary helpful information. In some cases, diets avoiding specific agents can be helpful in making a diagnosis and formal proof can be obtained using a double-blind placebo-controlled challenge. In general, and in contrast to many patients' belief, items in the diet are only a rare cause of severe, chronic asthma, although specific proven allergens, such as peanuts, shellfish, etc., can certainly cause acute bronchospasm as part of a generalised allergic reaction.

Stephen Durham

Dr Stephen R. Durham, MA, MD, FRCP, is Reader in Allergy and Clinical Immunology and Honorary Consultant Chest Physician at the Royal Brompton Hospital, London.

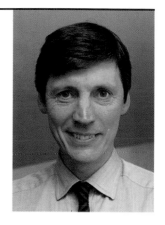

18
When should an asthma patient be referred to an allergist?

Allergists and organ-based physicians with an interest in allergy deal with "itch/sneeze/cough and wheeze". Their field of interest includes particularly summer hay fever, perennial rhinitis, allergic asthma, allergy to stinging insects, allergy-related skin disorders, drug allergy, food allergy and intolerance and anaphylaxis.

Many patients with asthma, particularly the young and middle aged are "atopic", which means that they manifest positive skin prick tests to common inhaled allergens. Atopy refers to a predisposition to develop allergic (IgE antibody mediated) diseases, including many of those listed above which are likely to be encountered frequently in the routine management of asthmatic patients.

Allergy should be managed in general practice by the GP or specialist practice nurse. Assessment of the importance (or otherwise) of allergy in a patient's asthma depends upon a carefully taken history of potential allergic triggers, particularly perennial allergens such as house dust mite and pets. Skin prick tests to the common allergens—cats, dogs, house dust mite and grass pollen—should, in my view, be performed in the routine assessment of all asthma patients. If there is concordance between the history and skin prick tests, the management is straightforward. Thus if the history and skin prick tests are both negative, no allergy-specific treatment is indicated. If the history and skin tests are positive, then careful consideration should be   39 given to recommending allergen avoidance measures in addition to conventional pharmacotherapy for asthma. Where there is "discordance", i.e., negative history with positive skin tests or positive history with negative skin tests, then a further more detailed history should be taken. If doubt remains, the patient should be referred to a routine NHS Allergy Clinic for further assessment, which might include further history taking, a wider panel of skin tests and, occasionally, allergen provocation tests. All patients with suspected occupational asthma should be referred for specialist assessment. Occupations "at risk" include paint-sprayers (isocyanates), solderers (colophony), laboratory workers (laboratory animal allergy) and health workers (latex, antibiotic allergy).

Food allergy, although more common in young children, is a rare cause of asthma exacerbations in adults, particularly in the absence of other features of food allergy such as rash, buccal symptoms, itching, gastrointestinal symptoms or, rarely, anaphylaxis. If doubt remains, the patient should see an allergy specialist. I believe that all patients with anaphylaxis due to food, venom, drug or unidentified cause should be seen by an allergist for advice regarding self-injection with adrenaline and, where appropriate, should also receive advice from the dietician. Patients who develop venom anaphylaxis should be carefully considered for allergen injection immunotherapy. Also, although immunotherapy is not indicated for asthma, patients with severe summer hay fever unresponsive to topical therapy and antihistamines may also benefit from allergen injection immunotherapy. Patients with non-specific or polysymptomatic illness who frequently consider allergy may be important in their symptoms may also benefit from specialist referral, if only to exclude allergy in the majority of cases.

Bill Frankland

Dr A.W. Frankland, DM, FRCP, is Honorary
Consulting Allergist at Guy's Hospital, London.

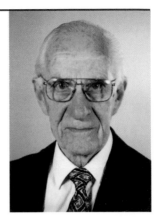

19

**What are the most common allergens which can cause anaphylaxis in
the asthma patient and what is the treatment?**

Although drugs and particularly penicillin are the most frequently implicated agents causing anaphylaxis, there is no good evidence that the allergic
asthmatic is especially likely to be sensitised anaphylactically to drugs. The
asthmatic, however, may be frequently treated with antibiotics and for this
reason is more liable eventually to become sensitised.

The next most common cause of IgE mediated anaphylaxis is hymenoptera (bee and wasp) stings. Asthmatic patients do not seem to have an
increased risk of developing systemic reactions to hymenoptera stings but
they do show significantly more severe reactions manifested by acute dys-
pnoea. The natural history of venom allergy is difficult to predict because up
to 40% of patients who have had a previous generalised reaction have no
reaction to a challenge sting. The rapidity of onset of symptoms, the severity
of symptoms, the patient's occupation and age and whether he or she is an
asthmatic are the most useful treatment guides.

Latex allergy has recently been increasing but unfortunately often goes
uninvestigated. Dentists, surgeons, nurses, housewives who wear rubber
gloves and children with spina bifida or hydrocephalus who have had many
operations are particularly liable to be sensitised. But in the atopic child who
uses a dummy and is not breast fed, latex allergy is met at an early age and
may give rise to anaphylactic sensitivity. Any patient with a known IgE   41

response to latex must always warn any dentist, anaesthetist and particularly surgeon of this. Fifteen patients died of latex anaphylaxis in the USA in 1995. Associated with latex allergy is quite often acute anaphylaxis to avocado pear, banana, chestnut and occasionally other fruit. A girl aged 18 died of banana anaphylaxis in the UK in 1996.

Foods are a more common cause of anaphylactic deaths in the UK than hymenoptera stings. Food allergy to eggs, milk and wheat are commonly seen in the atopic wheezy infant. Usually, these food allergies are outgrown but very occasionally a fish or egg sensitivity may persist through life. An allergy to nuts, particularly peanuts, that causes acute anaphylaxis usually persists through life. In a study of 1000 patients with nut anaphylaxis the first allergic reaction occurred in 60% of patients before the age of two years. One half had been admitted to hospital for treatment of anaphylaxis. Many infants had multiple food as well as multiple nut allergic reactions. Peanuts caused seven deaths in the UK in 1991–95, but brazil and cashew nuts also caused deaths. It is noteworthy that all the peanut deaths were in asthmatics. Six out of the seven, although they knew they were allergic to peanuts, did not realise they were at risk of dying and ate a food containing peanuts by mistake. Although upper airway obstruction causing stridor is very common in food anaphylaxis, it is lower airway obstruction causing asthma that gives rise to severe anaphylaxis and deaths in the asthmatic.

Treatment of anaphylaxis is by adrenaline. This must be given as soon as possible after the onset of the reaction. For adults the dosage is 0.3–1 mg of adrenaline 1 in 1000 given intramuscularly. For children the dose is 0.01 µg/kg. Patients at risk of anaphylaxis should have available their own pre-filled automatic adrenaline syringe. The Anapen or the Epipen auto-injector delivers a 0.3 mg dose of adrenaline which is given into the outer thigh. A child's version contains 0.15 mg of adrenaline. Syringes have a shelf life of two years. The Medihaler-Epi is a metered dose inhaler that delivers 280 µg adrenaline per puff. In children under the age of two years, three to five puffs are required. In older children 10 to 15 puffs and for an adult at least 20 puffs are required for a systemic effect. It must be remembered that an asthmatic may react biphasically so that two or three injections of adrenaline are required to maintain an adequate airway. All asthmatics should be given 100 mg of hydrocortisone intramuscularly or intravenously after the adrenaline. If there is much urticaria, intramuscular or intravenous injection of chloramphenamine is also needed. Blood pressure and peak flow should be monitored every 15 minutes. If there is no quick response to treatment, oxygen on the way to hospital by ambulance must be given to all asthmatics.

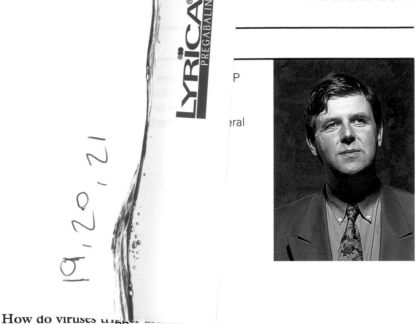

P

ʒral

How do viruses trigg~~

Acute respiratory infections, commonly with viruses, are the most frequent human illness. A range of viruses can be implicated, from influenza and para-influenza viruses to rhinoviruses and respiratory syncytial virus (RSV) infection. While RSV infection is a common cause of wheezing in small children, in older children and adults the epidemiological evidence implicates the rhinovirus as being most relevant to asthma exacerbations. The rhinoviruses are a major cause of the common cold. The mechanism whereby viral infection, and in particular rhinoviral infection, affects the airways has been studied in both normal and asthmatic subjects.

Within the upper airways, rhinoviral infection starts in the nose and spreads to the throat, infecting the most superficial lining cells (the epithelium). Once in these cells the viruses replicate, this process peaking about 48 hours after the initial inoculation, and can remain present for up to three weeks. Infection of the cells induces an inflammatory host response to rid the body of infected cells. This involves the shedding of epithelial cells and the release of mediators, in particular ones called kinins and prostaglandins. These mediators, through their direct actions on blood vessels and mucous glands or by their indirect effects via nerve stimulation, can be implicated in the development of nasal obstruction, runny nose, sore throat and cough. These mediators also have the potential to induce bronchospasm, particularly in the presence of "twitchy" airways as occurs in asthma. 43

Potentially more important, however, for the induction of the chest tightness and breathlessness associated with virus infection and for the fall in lung function, is the identification that viral infection induces eosinophil recruitment within the lower airways. This occurs in all subjects but the eosinophils are present within the airways for longer in asthma, so the chest problems take longer to "throw off" and, on account of the allergic inflammation within the airways, the eosinophils in asthma will have a heightened state of activation. Activated eosinophils release mediators, in particular leukotrienes, which are very potent at constricting the airways and inducing secretion of mucus.

So it is through the viral infection of epithelial cells that there is worsening of the eosinophilic airway inflammation in asthma and a clinical deterioration in asthma control. As epithelial shedding can continue for weeks and the physiological consequences may take four to eight weeks to recover fully in the absence of intervention, the sooner treatment is increased to limit the airway inflammation the quicker the recovery. At present it is impossible to avoid viral colds completely but it is hoped that vaccines may be developed in the future, such as those currently available for influenza. As influenza has similar or potentially more severe effects than rhinoviral infections, it is recommended that asthmatics receive prophylactic influenza vaccination to limit the effects of any such infection.

Mike Morgan

Dr Michael D.L. Morgan, MD, FRCP, is
Consultant Physician in Respiratory Medicine at
Glenfield Hospital, Leicester.

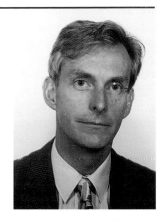

21
How does exercise trigger asthma?

Physical activity may trigger symptoms in the majority of people who suffer
from asthma. However, the health benefits and pleasure derived from
exercise should not be denied to sufferers and this particular trigger factor
should be managed rather than be avoided. Exercise of reasonable intensity
normally results in a minor degree of bronchodilation in normal subjects
and those with asthma. In approximately 80% of patients with asthma,
bronchoconstriction will result from six minutes of reasonably intense
exercise. This is manifest as a fall in forced expiratory volume in the first
second of expiration (FEV_1) or peak expiratory flow (PEF), to below 10 or
15% of baseline, which occurs 5 to 10 minutes after the end of exercise and
recovers by 30 to 40 minutes. Some patients may additionally have a late
response some hours later. The symptom of exercise-induced asthma (EIA)
characteristically continues for some time after the activity has ceased, which
distinguishes it from other causes of exertional breathlessness. A second
exercise challenge within 12 hours of the first may demonstrate a refractory
period. Some forms of exercise, such as swimming, appear to be less pro-
vocative than running or cycling. However, when corrected for work
intensity and climatic condition, there may be little difference.

There is still some debate about the exact nature of EIA. The trigger is
thought to be the hyperventilation of exercise, which results in cooling and
drying of the airways following the failure of the normal nasal conditioning 45

of inspired air. According to the most popular theory, osmotic changes induced by drying of the airway lining fluid subsequently triggers mediator release and bronchospasm. An alternative but less plausible theory implicates bronchial vascular hyperaemia as the mechanism and effector of bronchial obstruction. The sensitivity of the asthmatic individual to exercise challenge may be preconditioned by previous instability, allergen challenge or even atmospheric pollution exposure.

In some patients with asthma, exercise-induced symptoms may be the only manifestation of the condition and therefore the principles of treatment may have to be modified. As well as the usual emphasis on prevention, treatment should be aimed at modifying the trigger where possible and pre-medicating with short or long acting bronchodilator or cromoglycate as determined by individual experiment. For the serious athlete, changes in training or competition patterns to take advantage of the refractory period may also be helpful.

In spite of the fact that physical exercise adversely affects patients with asthma it should not be discouraged. Exercise intolerance in patients with asthma is still more likely to be due to lack of physical fitness than the limiting effects of the disease. This may result either from inadequate recognition and treatment or from the fear that exercise is harmful. Most patients with asthma who are correctly treated should be capable of normal physical activity and should be encouraged to participate.

Chapter 2

Paediatric Asthma: Issues, diagnosis, treatment and management

Andrew Bush

Dr Andrew Bush, MB BS (Hons), MA, MD, FRCP, is Senior Lecturer in Paediatric Respiratory Medicine at the National Heart and Lung Institute, Imperial College of Science, Technology and Medicine, London, and Honorary Consultant Paediatric Chest Physician at the Royal Brompton Hospital, London.

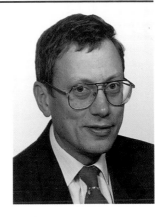

22
Do children grow out of asthma?

The definition of asthma that I shall use is clinical: recurrent episodes of cough and/or wheeze, in the absence of any other underlying diagnosis. This is important, because different groups mean different things by the label "asthma", for example labelling infants who wheeze only with colds as "virus associated wheeze". Thus my answer is really to the question, do recurrently wheezy children ever stop having episodes of wheeze?

The most quoted study of children with early onset wheeze comes from Tucson, but the conclusions of an (excellent) study in the heat of the desert where cockroaches rather than house dust mite are the commonest allergen should not be applied uncritically to more temperate climes. In Tucson, about half of all children wheeze at some time in the first six years of life. Two thirds of those who wheeze in the first three years of life will be symptom free at age six. Half of those wheezing at age six (which is about a third of the total population of six year olds) will have had persistent wheeze from the first three years of life, the other half will have wheezed for the first time after their third birthday. Those most likely to be in the symptom free category wheeze with colds but not at other times, and do not have a personal or family history of atopy. There is some evidence that these infants may be more susceptible to chronic obstructive pulmonary disease in mid to late adulthood. However, even atopic infants who wheeze may have a 50% chance of outgrowing their symptoms, at least temporarily. This group

49

contains some of those with the best prognosis (non-atopic wheezers with colds) and some of the worst (those with early onset atopy and a family history of asthma). Predictions are particularly difficult in this age group.

The pattern of symptoms in older children may be rather different. For obvious reasons, there is a dearth of good long-term prospective studies of asthma prognosis. Prospective studies of asthma in children aged seven to nine have shown that 20 years later, around two thirds will be symptom free. Various different symptom patterns have been shown; some children, in particular those with mild symptoms in adolescence and good lung function, will go into sustained remission. Nearly three quarters of those with infrequent symptoms at age 14 were virtually asymptomatic at age 28. Others have persistent ongoing symptoms; two thirds of those with frequent wheeze at age 14 were still symptomatic at age 28. Other possible risk factors for ongoing asthma include a personal history of atopy, fixed airflow obstruction, female sex and a history of asthma in the parents. A third group appear to go into remission, only to relapse in adulthood. Even 20 year prospective studies do not provide the complete answer; follow-up for many decades more may show that many children have only had a temporary remission.

Most of the parents who ask if children grow out of asthma are interested not in scientific prospective data, but whether their own child will outgrow his or her asthma. The answer has to be a resounding "maybe". It is difficult to make individual predictions, whatever the age of the child. If there has been no improvement by puberty, however, then complete remission is unlikely. Overall, an encouraging prognosis is justified, tempered with increasing caution for more severe symptoms in the atopic child. However, even for the child asymptomatic on no treatment, a relapse is possible, and probably the child will never lose the potential to wheeze. What remains to be seen is whether the early and aggressive use of anti-inflammatory agents will improve the prognosis for groups which would have been considered high risk 20 years ago.

Jon Couriel

Dr Jon Couriel, MA, FRCP, is Consultant in
Paediatric Respiratory Medicine at Booth Hall
Children's Hospital, Manchester.

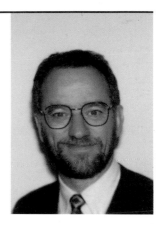

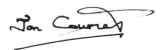

23
What effect does adult smoking have on childhood asthma?

Many parents of children with asthma ask if environmental factors worsen
or cause their child's symptoms. Concerns about traffic pollution, about
pets, about diet, and about how they can best reduce exposure to house
dust mite, are common. Unfortunately, many parents are reluctant to
accept that their smoking affects their child's asthma—"but we never
smoke in front of the children, doctor" is a frequent response to questions
on the subject. And yet, as a recent large National Asthma Campaign survey
has shown, 74% of asthmatic children believe smoky places make their
asthma worse.

Between a third and a half of asthmatic children in Britain live in a home
where at least one adult smokes cigarettes. Analysis of the urine or saliva of
children exposed to smoke shows they absorb significant amounts of
nicotine and other toxic chemicals. We have known for over 20 years that
children of parents who smoke are at increased risk of serious respiratory
illnesses such as bronchiolitis and pneumonia and of other chest symptoms.
The more cigarettes the parents smoke at home, the greater the effect on
the child. Maternal smoking is more important than paternal smoking and
infants are more susceptible than older children. If parents smoke, their
children are more likely to take up smoking themselves.

Children with asthma are particularly sensitive to environmental tobacco
smoke. Many studies have shown that these children have more frequent

51

and severe symptoms, an earlier onset of asthma, greater use of asthma medications, and poorer lung function if their parents, and particularly if their mother, smokes. Even more worrying is the growing body of evidence that maternal smoking in pregnancy impairs the growth and development of the unborn infant's lungs.

Several prospective studies of the factors which influence lung development have shown that babies born to mothers who smoke through the pregnancy have smaller, more reactive, airways than the infants of non-smoking mothers. Perhaps not surprisingly, these babies with smaller airways are much more likely to suffer repeated respiratory symptoms, such as wheeze, cough and breathlessness, than are control infants. These effects persist for many years and are most evident in children with a family history of atopic disease. As 38% of women in this country smoke regularly in early pregnancy, and only a quarter of these quit, the implications of these findings are serious.

All of us need to recognise that parental smoking—an important and avoidable burden on the health of many children—is particularly detrimental to children who have, or are at risk of developing, asthma. We must inform parents who smoke that their smoking will be having a harmful effect on their child's asthma. We need to offer support and practical advice for those who want to quit smoking, rather than chastising them. And we need to be less defeatist about this issue: perhaps a first small step would be to stop talking euphemistically about "passive smoking" and start calling it "involuntary smoking".

Mark Levy

Dr Mark L. Levy, MB ChB, FRCGP, is a General Practitioner in Harrow, Middlesex, a past Chairman of the GPs in Asthma Group and the Medical Adviser of the National Asthma Training Centre.

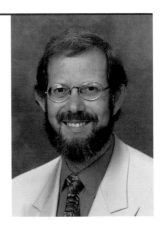

24

How can under- and over-diagnosis of asthma in children in primary care be avoided?

Under-diagnosis of childhood asthma may lead to many years of misery and frustration affecting the whole family, as well as the danger that children may not regain their optimum lung function if left untreated. The danger of over-diagnosis is coupled with the risk of over-treatment and therefore we should try and be as precise as possible when diagnosing asthma in children. Peer group audit or local awareness of the prevalence of childhood asthma is helpful in determining whether a practice's diagnosis of asthma is above or below average. In the early 1980s the prevalence of diagnosed childhood asthma was under 5%. Now, in 1997, as a result of heightened awareness within primary care, there are concerns that the condition may be "over-diagnosed". Recent National Asthma Training Centre data confirmed a very wide spectrum of the prevalence of diagnosed asthma in children born in 1987; ranging from 0 to over 30% (mean 12.3%) in 466 UK general practices caring for over three million patients. Therefore it is possible that asthma currently is both under- and over-diagnosed, depending on various factors.

First let us consider how to avoid under-diagnosing childhood asthma. This can be achieved by maintaining a heightened awareness of possible asthma. Sometimes, a child presents with very obvious asthma symptoms and most clinicians would have little difficulty in making a diagnosis. 53

However, there are still considerable delays in diagnosing many children and we need to be aware of the clues that should arouse our suspicions. For example, the presence, in the NHS records, of frequent consultations for respiratory symptoms, allergy or eczema, or a family history of asthma or allergy that indicates that a child is at risk for developing asthma. By adopting a practice policy of numbering all respiratory consultations from birth onwards, the primary care team would soon become aware that a child possibly has asthma. Strong indications of childhood asthma in the records include: more than three respiratory consultations per year; more than three episodes of wheezing combined with a family history of atopy; family members who smoke; the presence of pets (especially cats) in the home; and respiratory symptoms exacerbated by exercise, laughter or viral infections.

Confirmation of asthma is difficult in young children (under five years); we have to rely on the personal and family history coupled with evidence of a response to appropriate therapy. However, since asthma is a condition typically involving recurrent episodes it is difficult to be sure whether a child's symptoms have resolved naturally or as a result of the therapy! The availability of objective measurements (peak expiratory flow) enables us to confirm the diagnosis in older children by demonstrating reversible airflow obstruction.

Now let us turn to how to avoid over-diagnosing childhood asthma. Failure to distinguish between brief episodic symptoms and chronic persisting asthma may result in over-diagnosis and over-treatment of asthma. Those children who present with episodic symptoms, perhaps associated with viral infections, may need to be treated simply with short courses of therapy rather than diagnosed as chronic asthmatics and then treated continuously with prophylaxis.

In the absence of an objective test for asthma in very young children, it may be wise to review the diagnosis at regular intervals. While it would be a retrograde step to re-introduce the term "wheezy bronchitis", which contributed to delays in asthma diagnosis and treatment in the last decade, it is perhaps time for us to reconsider our use of the term "asthma". If asthma is suspected, perhaps we should enter the words "possible asthma" or "unconfirmed asthma" in the records, thereby avoiding the danger of missing the diagnosis, while maintaining awareness of its possible existence in children. The diagnosis can be reviewed at a later date when the child presents with new symptoms. Stepping down the treatment in asthmatic children who are asymptomatic, in association with peak flow diaries (if the child is old enough), may be helpful in identifying children no longer in need of continuous therapy.

Clear, validated, protocols for use of the term "asthma" and for subsequent review of the diagnosis in children are required. A task for the future?

Mike Silverman

Professor Michael Silverman, MA, MD, DCH, FRCP, is Professor of Child Health and Head of the Department of Child Health at the University of Leicester.

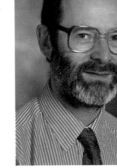

25
How is asthma diagnosed in the under twos?

There is no consensus about the use of the term "asthma" in very young children. Many terms were formerly used to name wheezing diseases in the very young but, with the advent of effective bronchodilator and preventer therapy, these terms were superseded by the label "asthma", in order to encourage doctors to use appropriate therapy. It is now clear that, in the pre-school age group, there are several syndromes whose common feature, recurrent or variable wheezing, would reasonably allow the term "asthma" to be used. These syndromes include: wheezing disease in an atopic child, or with a family history of atopy; discrete episodes of wheeze and cough associated with viral upper respiratory tract infections, often independent of atopy; wheezing associated with pre-term birth; and wheezing associated with gastro-oesophageal reflux.

I believe that it is important to differentiate between types of asthma in under twos. The long-term prognosis (at school age and later) is better for those children who are non-atopic, with a negative maternal history of asthma, from a non-smoking family, and who only have episodes of wheeze associated with viral infection. The prognosis is likely to be worse (i.e., persistent atopic asthma is more probable) if there is strong personal and family history of atopy and persistent wheeze between viral infections brought about by trigger factors such as exercise, laughter, allergic agents, smoke and strong smells. Another reason for differentiating is that children 55 with purely episodic viral wheeze may respond less effectively to preventer treatment with inhaled corticosteroids than do those with persistent wheeze between episodes.

The cardinal feature in the diagnosis of asthma is history of variable wheeze, almost always associated with cough. While expiratory wheeze and dry cough are typical of older children, in young children during exacerbations a moist or "rattly" cough is often found, sometimes associated with mucous vomiting. The wheeze itself, although typically expiratory, is often difficult to characterise, particularly in acute severe airway obstruction when an important differential diagnosis is stridor (or inspiratory sound). The variable nature of the associated breathing difficulties (and of difficulty speaking and feeding), the variety of trigger factors and the fact that there may be no sign at all during physical examination, mean that careful history taking is of the utmost importance. During an acute exacerbation, obvious signs of distress, chest hyper-inflation, indrawing of the lower ribs on inspiration and the use of accessory muscles of breathing are all clues to the presence of airway obstruction. Obvious cyanosis suggests life-threatening obstruction.

A daily record card (diary card) is a useful means of recording day-to-day symptoms in order to confirm variability. It can also be used to demonstrate a therapeutic response in the home environment. There is no diagnostic test which would confirm the presence of asthma. Observations such as allergy tests and tests for gastro-oesophageal reflux can provide clues to the cause while oximetry will provide information about the severity of airway obstruction.

In school-age children, a response to an adequate dose of an inhaled bronchodilator is a confirmatory test for asthma. A similar therapeutic trial can be carried out in pre-school children. During a wheezy episode, give either a nebulised dose of salbutamol or terbutaline (2.5 or 5 mg respectively) or five to 10 puffs of salbutamol by metered-dose inhaler/spacer/face mask, and observe the child over the next 15 minutes. The resolution of symptoms strongly suggests a diagnosis of asthma and this can be confirmed by a longer therapeutic trial at home.

Probably the most certain method of diagnosis is to await the outcome of wheezing disease. As school age approaches it becomes increasingly clear which children have classical atopic asthma and which have transient pre-school viral episodic wheeze. Until this happens, however, it is as well to use the general label "asthma" to describe all these conditions, but to explain to parents the variety of conditions which falls under the heading and to give them some idea of the likely prognosis based on the pattern of disease exhibited by their own children.

David Heaf

Dr David Heaf, MB, BS, FRCP, is Consultant
Paediatrician (Respiratory Medicine) at the Royal
Liverpool Children's NHS Trust-Alder Hey.

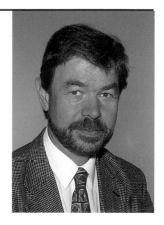

26
How is recurrent wheezing managed in the under twos?

Over 20% of children wheeze before the age of two. Less than half of these children are likely to have asthma or respond to asthma treatment. Recurrent wheeze can be due to small airways, often related to the mother smoking in pregnancy, viral infections such as respiratory syncytial virus (RSV) bronchiolitis as well as early asthma. A history can often distinguish between the different causes of wheeze and so guide management. A constant wheeze, with no wheeze free period, indicates fixed airway narrowing and requires referral. Episodic wheeze, with acute episodes only, is often due to viral infections and responds poorly to regular asthma treatment. Interval wheeze, with symptoms between acute episodes, is most likely to respond to asthma treatment. A family history of atopy, especially in the mother, or eczema in the child would support the diagnosis of early asthma.

In the under twos a four to eight week trial of asthma treatment is the most useful diagnostic test. A diary card can be used to record symptom improvement. Treatment should be stopped if there is a poor response, and an alternative cause for recurrent wheeze should be sought.

As with older patients the inhaled route is the best way of delivering asthma treatment in the under twos. The large volume spacer and mask can be used to deliver all types of treatment and a home nebuliser is rarely necessary. The child patient's carers need careful instruction and patience if treatment is to be effective.

β_2 agonists have been shown to be effective under the age of two years and are the reliever treatment of choice. Ipratropium bromide (Atrovent) may be an effective alternative. Regular preventive therapy should be started in any patient who is getting interval symptoms or acute episodes more than every two to four weeks. Sodium cromoglycate does not appear to be as effective in this age group as it is in older children and inhaled corticosteroids are the preventer treatment of choice. The dose of inhaled corticosteroid has to be relatively large because of the inefficient delivery devices. A starting dose of 100 to 200 mcg twice daily of beclomethasone or budesonide should be used initially to demonstrate effectiveness. However, this dose could be reduced if symptoms are controlled, and the lowest dose that achieves control should be used.

More work needs to be done to demonstrate which measures may reduce the development of chronic childhood asthma. Reducing house dust mite load may be important but diet is probably not. However, there is no doubt that preventing exposure to cigarette smoke before and after birth will have a significant effect on the recurrent wheeze.

Peter Weller

Dr Peter H. Weller, MA, MB BChir, FRCP, is
Consultant Paediatrician (Respiratory Medicine)
at Birmingham Children's and City Hospitals,
Birmingham.

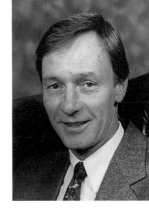

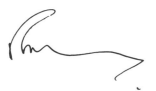

27
How is an acute attack of childhood asthma managed?

An acute attack of asthma in childhood classically presents as wheezing, cough and breathlessness, although sometimes the wheezing is not obvious. It can be the first presentation of asthma, especially in a pre-school child in relation to a viral infection, or an exacerbation in a child known to have asthma.

Acute severe asthma presents with acute breathlessness and wheeze, with inability to talk and hypoxaemia. Peak flow is likely to be unrecordable in those old enough to perform the test. In a very severe attack the chest can be almost silent, with marked hyper-inflation. Immediate treatment is required with oxygen, nebulised β_2 agonists and systemic corticosteroids, with admission to hospital for further treatment and monitoring.

A moderate attack presents with wheeze and cough, symptoms sometimes being more obvious than signs in the chest. A reliable peak flow reading can be helpful in the older child (over seven years) and heart rate is an important objective measure of severity. Both can be useful in monitoring response to treatment. Inhaled β_2 agonists, either via a nebuliser or a similar dose by a large volume spacer, are given, together with an oral corticosteroid (e.g., soluble prednisolone 0.5–1.0 mgm/kg per dose), given for three to five days. The β_2 agonist will need to be repeated every two to four hours and the response to treatment monitored either in the surgery or at home. If there is no response to the inhaled   59 treatment or if it has to be repeated within two hours, hospital admission should be considered.

It is common practice to double inhaled treatment at the first sign of a viral infection. If cough or wheeze are persisting or increasing despite increased treatment, including regular bronchodilators, a short course of soluble prednisolone (0.5–1.0 mgm/kg per dose) given early for three days, can prevent a more severe exacerbation. These short courses are safe even if required three to four times a year.

After recovery the need for prophylactic treatment needs to be assessed, together with a simple action plan to be instigated at the first signs of a further exacerbation.

Katharine King

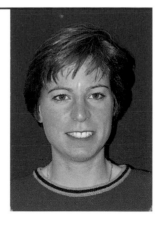

Dr Katharine J. King, MBBS, MRCGP, DRCOG, is a General Practitioner in Stratford-upon-Avon, Warwickshire. She is Clinical Assistant in Respiratory Medicine at Warwick Hospital and Medical Lecturer at the National Asthma Training Centre.

28
What is the ideal dosage regime for oral corticosteroids in children?

Children with asthma may need oral corticosteroids in order to attain control in an acute attack, at any step in the management of chronic asthma or occasionally as part of their regular management in severe disease.

The usual regime in an acute attack is 1–2 mg prednisolone per kg body weight (maximum 40 mg) for up to five days. There is no need to taper the dose of corticosteroid when using these short, sharp courses. The child should be reassessed in 24 to 48 hours and admitted to hospital if there is no significant improvement. Prednisolone is available in a soluble form to aid administration. Vomiting is common in children and a dose should be repeated if this occurs within one hour. Response to treatment should be monitored closely by parents and doctors. Parents should be encouraged to assess their child's progress and can usually decide when to stop treatment. Once the child is old enough to monitor peak flows, an objective measure of progress can be obtained. Otherwise, such markers as quality of sleep, persistence of cough or wheeze and exercise related symptoms are good indicators. After a course of oral corticosteroids, overall management needs re-evaluating in order to try and prevent further attacks.

In chronic asthma it is sometimes beneficial to use a short course of oral corticosteroids whatever step in treatment the child is on in order to re-establish stability. This has the advantages of getting the child well quickly (and so minimising sleepless nights, time off school, etc.) as well as fully suppressing residual airway inflammation so that inhaled therapy can work more effectively. The same dosage regime as for an acute attack can be used although 1 mg prednisolone per kg body weight is often sufficient. The duration of treatment should be kept to the minimum necessary to achieve the desired results.

The use of regular oral corticosteroids is fortunately rare in children. Some asthmatics who remain uncontrolled on high dose inhaled corticosteroids and bronchodilators including nebulized β_2 antagonists and/or slow release xanthines (if tolerated) do need the addition of alternate day low dose (5–10 mg) prednisolone. By using alternate day regimes, the effects on the hypothalamus pituitary adrenal (HPA) axis and long-term side effects are reduced. Children receiving such treatment will usually be under a paediatric specialist who will closely monitor and review their continuing need for treatment.

In summary, oral corticosteroids are an important part of the management armoury in childhood asthma. The dose used is 1–2 mg prednisolone per kg body weight (maximum 40 mg) and the duration of treatment is usually one to five days. Rarely, regular corticosteroids are necessary and where possible in such cases an alternate day regime should be used.

Søren Pedersen

Professor Søren Pedersen, MD, is Professor at the University of Odense and Department of Paediatrics, Kolding Hospital, DK-6000 Kolding, Denmark.

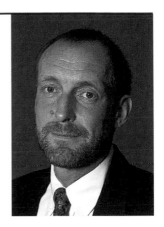

29
What are the benefits of inhaled corticosteroid therapy in children?

Inhaled corticosteroids affect a variety of clinical outcome measures. A drug may control one outcome parameter, such as symptoms, without having any effects upon other outcomes, such as airway hyper-responsiveness or acute exacerbations. Therefore, it is important to chose a treatment that influences as many outcome parameters as possible. Inhaled corticosteroids have significant and often marked beneficial effects upon a large variety of outcome parameters, including reduction in symptoms, improvement in lung function, reduction in frequency and severity of acute exacerbations, reduction in mortality and morbidity, improvement in quality of life, cost-effectiveness, control of airway hyper-responsiveness, normalisation of the chronic inflammatory changes in the airways, prevention of airway remodelling and normal growth of lung function. Furthermore, inhaled corticosteroids are effective in patients with asthma regardless of disease severity. By comparison, chronic treatment with all other asthma drugs influences fewer outcome parameters, having mainly been shown in controlled trials to have a significant reproducible effect upon symptoms and lung function.

Low doses of inhaled corticosteroids are very effective. The vast majority of children will achieve optimal symptom control and effect on peak expiratory flow rates, and a marked effect on the other outcome parameters, at daily doses of less than 400 µg/day.

The beneficial effects of inhaled corticosteroids are more pronounced than for any other anti-asthma drug (sodium cromoglycate, nedocromil sodium, theophylline and long-acting β_2 agonists, as shown in a number of studies. In recent studies, children with mild and moderate asthma achieved markedly better symptom control, significantly higher morning and evening peak expiratory flow rates and clinical lung function during treatment with 50 µg fluticasone propionate twice daily, as compared with children treated with sodium cromoglycate 20 mg four times daily. So far, no controlled clinical studies have found other drugs to be more effective than inhaled corticosteroids in children with asthma.

Furthermore, early treatment with inhaled corticosteroids appears to be advantageous. The improvement in lung function seems to be greater and the control of symptoms better in children who start treatment with inhaled corticosteroids early (within 2 years) after the onset of asthma than in children who do not start the treatment until some years after onset of asthma symptoms. Also, children who start inhaled corticosteroids early require lower doses to maintain asthma control. Early use also reduces the risk of under-treatment.

The overall picture is thus as follows. Inhaled corticosteroids have been used for the treatment of asthma in children for more than 20 years. During this time, a substantial number of studies have been performed evaluating the safety and efficacy of this therapy. Generally, the results have been reassuring. In patients with mild and moderate asthma, low daily doses of around 100–200 µg/day of inhaled corticosteroid produce a clinical effect which, in most trials, is better than the effect of any other treatment to which it has been compared. No clinically important side effects have been associated with treatment in this dose range. Inhaled corticosteroids beneficially affect more outcome parameters than any other anti-asthma drug. Furthermore, early intervention with inhaled corticosteroids facilitates, and may be a pre-condition for, long-term optimal asthma control. The marked efficacy and many beneficial effects of low doses of inhaled corticosteroids, combined with the lack of clinically important systemic side effects, give this treatment a favourable benefit/risk ratio compared with other treatments. This supports placing this treatment as a first-line therapy in children with asthma requiring a continuous prophylactic treatment. Since the occurrence of measurable systemic effects increases with dose, the lowest dose which controls the disease should always be used.

John Price

Professor John F. Price, MA, MD, FRCP, is
Professor of Paediatric Respiratory Medicine and
Head of the Academic Department of Child
Health at King's College Hospital, London.

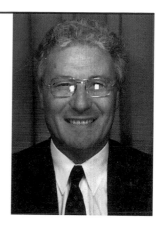

30
What risks are there for children taking inhaled corticosteroid therapy?

There appears to be individual, end organ and tissue variation in responsiveness to glucocorticoids. In some children, treatment with inhaled corticosteroid is associated with a reduction in daily cortisol excretion, and in short term growth of the lower leg. The threshold dose at which these systemic effects can be detected ranges from 400–800 mcg/day. Such effects become clinically relevant if the capacity of the adrenal gland to respond to stress is impaired or there is an adverse effect on bone metabolism or height velocity.

Urinary free cortisol is a useful guide to over-activity of the adrenal gland but a poor indicator of hypothalamus pituitary adrenal (HPA) axis suppression. Low morning plasma cortisol suggests adrenal suppression and the need to test the response to adrenocorticotropic hormone (ACTH). A stimulation test using 500 ng of synacthen is safer and more discriminating than one using 250 mcg.

The dynamics of bone turnover in children are different from adults. Biochemical and physical studies of bone metabolism in children are hampered by a lack of age and sex specific normal values. Osteocalcin is probably the marker of choice for bone formation and pyridinium collagen crosslinks for bone resorption. The results of short-term and cross-sectional studies have been inconsistent but one longitudinal study found a reduction in osteocalcin after 400–800 mcg/day of inhaled corticosteroid. The value 65 of densitometry in asthmatic children receiving inhaled corticosteroids is not yet established but the little data available suggest 300–400 mcg/day has no adverse effect on bone density.

Measurement of lower leg growth by knemometry is a valuable research technique particularly for comparing systemic adsorption with different inhaled corticosteroids. However the relationship between growth of the lower leg over a few weeks and long-term linear growth is not known. Linear growth velocity in asthmatic children is influenced by seasonal variation, delay in puberty, disease severity and the use of oral corticosteroids. These variables must be taken into account when assessing the effects of inhaled corticosteroids on growth. Height measurements made over less than one year are liable to misinterpretation.

There is no evidence that inhaled corticosteroids when appropriately prescribed in standard doses have any adverse effect on long-term growth. Growth deceleration has been recorded in children with very mild intermittent asthma given 400 mcg/day of inhaled corticosteroid. Some children with severe asthma taking inhaled corticosteroid in doses greater than 800 mcg/day show a decrease in height velocity; others on the other hand may show an increase in growth rate as the asthma becomes better controlled. Children taking high doses of inhaled corticosteroid should have their height measured using a stadiometer every three to four months. For reliable results both in research and in clinical practice the measurements should be done by trained personnel using regularly calibrated equipment.

When properly used, inhaled corticosteroids are extremely safe and the first priority must always be to treat the asthma adequately.

Carrie McKenzie

Dr Carrie McKenzie, MB ChB, MRCP, DCCH, MD, is Consultant Paediatrician and Medical Director at Sheffield Children's Hospital NHS Trust.

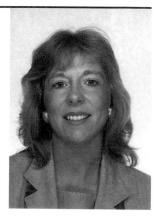

31
How important is the height measurement of asthmatic children and how should it be done?

Growth in childhood is the most natural of phenomena. The continuous process of height gain along expected channels on growth charts is an excellent indicator of general well-being.

Childhood growth can be subdivided into three distinct phases. First, a rapid but decelerating period of two to three years. Second, a period of steady growth at a relatively constant rate before the third phase, of the prepubertal lull in growth and then the massive growth spurt associated with the onset of puberty. Each phase is regulated by different factors, including nutrition, growth hormone and sex steroids.

Children with asthma may grow abnormally for a variety of reasons. The disease itself if unrecognised or under-treated may cause maturational delay with associated short stature. The precise mechanism of this growth delay is unknown. It is clear, however, that with appropriate management, children with asthma can be allowed to fulfil their genetic height potential.

The chronic use of oral corticosteroids causes permanent stunting, and the possible role of inhaled corticosteroids in growth suppression has been much debated in the literature. The emerging consensus of opinion is that treatment with inhaled beclomethasone or budesonide at doses of up to 800 mcg daily has no adverse effect on height. A new inhaled corticosteroid with negligible oral bioavailability, fluticasone propionate, has an improved safety profile. The accumulating evidence with this new drug is that in studies performed over one year there is no adverse effect on growth at doses up to 200 mcg daily.

There are, however, case reports in the literature of individuals who appear to suffer from marked growth suppression when treated with inhaled corticosteroids. This effect is reversible on cessation of treatment. These children appear to suffer from idiosyncratic responses which may be steroid specific. Some of these children have been successfully switched to an alternative inhaled corticosteroid compound and displayed impressive "catch-up growth".

Reports of studies investigating the interaction of asthma and its various treatments with growth are subject to a number of confounding factors, such as measurement error, compliance, disease severity, seasonal variation of growth rate, pubertal status and socio-economic factors.

Stadiometry provides an accurate, non-invasive clinical tool which is universally available, relatively inexpensive and demands little formal training on the part of the practitioner. In order to be a clinically relevant indicator of well-being, measurements of height must be performed by trained individuals using well-maintained, regularly calibrated equipment.

The accuracy of measurements is improved by using a single observer and ensuring that the child is positioned without shoes so that the heels and back are in contact with the vertical measuring column. Gentle but firm upwards pressure must be applied beneath the mastoid process to help the child stretch. The head must be positioned so that the lower border of the eye socket is in the same plane as the external auditory meatus. At each visit several individual height recordings should be made.

While stadiometry does not provide rapid answers, it can provide useful long-term information. Every child with asthma deserves wholly appropriate management and should have their height measured at least three times per year. Any significant deviations from expected growth patterns should be further investigated with the help of a paediatric endocrinologist.

Bill Holmes

Dr Bill Holmes, B Med Sci, BM, BS, MRCGP, is a
General Practitioner in Nottingham.

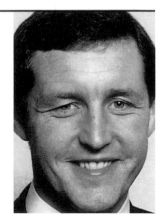

32
Is there any place for antibiotics in exacerbations of paediatric asthma?

In the words of H.I. Menken, American humorist: "For every complex
question, there is a simple answer, and it is usually wrong". Every illness is a
mixture of disease, temperament and circumstance. Asthma is no exception,
and when management addresses only one of these areas it is usually
inadequate and occasionally disastrous. For this reason, whether antibiotics
have a place in paediatric asthma is a complex question, for which a simple
answer—"no"—is clear but inadequate.

"Infection" as a cause for asthma (and, indeed, many other troubles) is
highly acceptable to parents and patients. It allows blame to be allocated
with impunity, and the concept that germs cause damage which resolves
when they are destroyed is easy to grasp; certainly very much easier than
understanding the mechanisms of inflammation. Parents usually welcome
courses of antibiotics—indeed, they are often perceived as markers of
thoroughness and care when in fact they may be neither. The pressure to
use antibiotics is considerable, and a decision to withhold them can be
fraught with trouble.

In the absence of acute respiratory distress few GPs would think it
unreasonable to use antibiotics in the management of a child presenting
with cough for the first time, even when asthma is being considered among
the differential diagnosis. There will be those who frown upon ever using
antibiotics in this situation, but many such consultations take place as 69

"emergencies" at the end of surgery, or out of hours, and a more leisurely consideration of the problem may be unrealistic. Denying anxious parents what they believe frequently to be necessary medication rarely forms the basis of a future successful relationship. Prescribing antibiotics in such circumstances may be reasonable, but at a cost. Antibiotics may rarely harm children, and they may buy some time, but when used to avoid the more time consuming and taxing task of addressing the diagnosis and treatment of asthma, they serve patients less well than they deserve, even if this is not something that is readily appreciated.

In chronic persistent asthma the problems arise, not with the initial prescription, but with the effect antibiotics have in reinforcing in the parents' mind an infective explanation for an inflammatory disorder. The consequences of this misunderstanding are considerable as parental cooperation is central to adherence to what may subsequently be long-term preventer therapy.

In acute severe asthma, most exacerbations are triggered by viruses. Antibiotics are therefore of no benefit, and are rarely indicated. Whilst it may be reasonable to bend a little from this standard when dealing with an acute problem, and while addressing broader issues in the consultation, the usual management of exacerbations should strictly adhere to appropriate anti-inflammatory and bronchodilator therapy.

Jeff Williams

Dr Jeff Williams, DCH, FRCP, is Consultant
Paediatrician at Glan Clwyd District General
Hospital NHS Trust, Rhyl, Denbighshire.

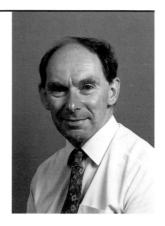

33
Do long acting β_2 agonists play a part in the management of children who have exercise-induced asthma?

Exercise and cold air induced symptoms are common in children with asthma and may inhibit normal play and sporting activity. It is likely that inflammation plays a substantial role and there is at least a transient increase in airway hyper-responsiveness. Severe exercise-induced asthma (EIA) can occur despite the presence of good basal lung function.

Regular treatment with inhaled corticosteroids reduces EIA but many children continue to have exercise-triggered symptoms even on moderately high doses of inhaled corticosteroids. Nevertheless, optimising inhaled corticosteroid dosage should be regarded as the first step in managing EIA. Cromones have also been shown to be effective when used prophylactically. The use of cromones in conjunction with inhaled corticosteroids has been recommended but means that an additional inhaler has to be taken to school which is both unwieldy and potentially confusing.

Treatment with oral agents, including β_2 agonists, theophylline containing drugs and antihistamines, have not been shown to be very effective in preventing exercise induced symptoms. The prophylactic use of short acting β_2 adrenoreceptor agonists delivered by aerosol immediately prior to exercise is very effective and has been a traditional recommendation. There are several drawbacks to this tactic. The duration of action is often less than two hours, the children must have their inhaler with them and must be

71

prepared to use it as well as remember to do so. Also much exercise in childhood is unpredictable. For these reasons the concept of using a long acting β_2 agonist is attractive.

Single dose studies using a long acting β_2 agonist have demonstrated significant protection against EIA for up to 12 hours. The precise mechanism by which this is accomplished is not yet clear. Certainly, prolonged bronchodilation occurs but there are other effects which may be relevant. These include inhibition of the bronchial responsiveness and both early and late bronchial reactions that follow allergen challenge. Some concern has been raised that the regular use of β_2 agonists might reduce overall control. Most studies have not confirmed this. However, a rational plan for persistent EIA in the face of appropriate inhaled corticosteroid treatment would be to administer a long acting β_2 agonist as a single daily dose in the morning. Depending on circumstances this might be a regular morning dose or tailored to pre-empt predictable activity.

Advice unrelated to drug treatment is also important. The manoeuvre of prolonged warm-up exercises may induce refractoriness to EIA without causing bronchoconstriction. This practice can be particularly recommended in instances such as competition sports where the child might be more able to comply. Lastly, it is important for children with asthma to avoid significant exercise during respiratory tract infections.

Paul McCarthy

Dr T. Paul McCarthy, MB, BS, MCPCH, MRCS, LRCP, DA, is the inventor of the McCarthy mask and lives in Bures Hamlet, Suffolk.

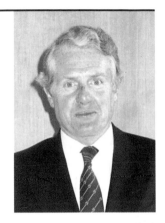

34
How is asthma treatment delivered to the under twos?

Health professionals agree that the preferred method of delivering asthma medication is by inhalation. As the drug is delivered directly to the lungs, lower doses can be used compared with the oral route. The risks of side effects are thereby reduced, and the onset of action may be expedited. The most commonly used inhalation devices are pressurised metered dose inhalers (PMDIs). Young children do not have the co-ordination needed to use PMDIs, but they may use large volume spacer devices that remove this need. The under twos rarely use these devices successfully. They are unlikely to close their lips around the mouthpiece and inhale, or may try to insert their tongues into the mouthpiece.

Since 1989 masks have been available that attach to spacer devices. It is now accepted that such a combination is the preferred method for delivery of asthma medication to children under two. To administer the drug, the device is tilted, with the mask end down, and the mask is applied to the child's face. The PMDI is activated, the drug flows through the device, and is inhaled by the child. If a seal between the mask and face is not achieved, the action of tilting the device opens the valve in the spacer. The mask should be closely applied to the face as any gap reduces the amount of drug inhaled. When corticosteroids are given, the child's face should be washed afterwards. For children who resist the application of a mask, it may be possible to administer the medication while the child is asleep. To familiarise 73 the child with the device and mask, he or she should be allowed to play with them. The parent may perhaps put a playbrick or toy inside so that they become a plaything. Any such toy should, of course, be removed before use.

In some cases, it may be necessary to use oral medication in the under twos, but the caveats regarding dosage, side effects and time of onset of action must be remembered. In acute severe asthma, glucocorticosteroids may be administered orally (or even by injection), but the inhaled therapy should be re-established as soon as possible.

Nebulisers are of use for this age group, especially in emergency situations. However, they should only be used for the administration of routine therapy where the child will not accept the spacer device and mask, as they are inconvenient, time-consuming and costly by comparison. In an emergency it may be possible to use a spacer device and mask instead of a nebuliser to deliver salbutamol or other therapy. An equivalent or smaller dose is used and administered one actuation at a time.

Devices suitable for the under twos include the Paediatric Volumatic and the Babyhaler (both Allen & Hanburys) and the Nebuhaler and Mask (Astra). With such devices both reliever and preventer therapy can be administered to the under twos. The instruction of the parent and child in their use may be time-consuming for the health professional, but the potential benefits in terms of asthma control, make it time well spent.

Emma Sergeant

Emma Sergeant RGN, RSCN, NATC Dip in
Asthma Care, is Head of Communications at the
National Asthma Training Centre.

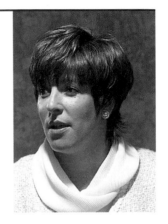

35
What are the appropriate delivery systems for children of different ages and why?

A common reason for failure of treatment is inappropriate selection or inappropriate use of an inhaler. Children rarely fit exactly into textbook categorisation but, for the purposes of selecting appropriate delivery systems for asthma treatments, pre school and school-age children form two distinct groups.

From birth to two years the most appropriate delivery system is a large volume spacer plus mask and a metered dose inhaler. This system does not require inspiratory coordination and a range of treatments can be delivered. The devices available include the Paediatric Volumatic (Laerdal mask), Nebuhaler with mask (McCarthy mask) and Babyhaler (Laerdal mask). Currently the Fisonair is not available with a mask in the United Kingdom.

Between the ages of three and four years a large volume spacer and metered dose inhaler are appropriate. Parents or carers will probably still need to help administer treatment. The child can tidal breathe through most of these devices (although not with the Fisonair) and can gradually be taught to breath hold in preparation for a device that is more portable.

From the age of five years most children can use breath-actuated devices. Inevitably some children will be able to use these devices sooner than others, and therefore review of inhaler technique on a regular basis is important at this stage. The available breath-actuated metered dose inhalers are the Autohaler and Easi-breathe devices, both of which contain β_2 agonists and inhaled corticosteroids. Dry powder devices available are the Spinhaler, Rotahaler, Diskhaler, Turbohaler and Accuhaler. The Spinhaler only delivers cromoglycate but the other devices deliver β_2 agonists and inhaled corticosteroids.

When selecting delivery devices for children it is important to consider the range of treatments available through the device; whether the device is loaded with multiple doses or whether it needs reloading; the amount of coordination needed to operate the device effectively; whether there is any way the child can tell how many doses are left in the device. With these factors in mind the health professional can select appropriate devices that meet the necessary criteria for an individual child. From this selection the child (and parent) can choose a device that they like. Patient involvement will aid compliance.

Once the selection of a new delivery device has been made it is vital to check that the child can use the device correctly and that the parent/child understands the treatment regimen. If the child requires high doses of inhaled corticosteroids it may still be appropriate for them to continue to use a large volume spacer and metered dose inhaler at home, with a more portable device for their medication.

Chris O'Callaghan

Dr Chris O'Callaghan, B Med Sci, BM, BS, FRCP, DM, MCPCH, is Consultant Paediatrician and Senior Lecturer in Child Health at the University of Leicester.

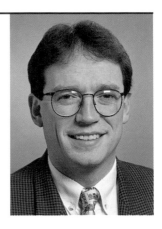

36
What are the technical issues around delivery systems for children?

Most aerosol drug devices were developed for adult patients and their use extrapolated to children. The initial drugs used in these systems were bronchodilators, and as extremely little drug is required for maximum bronchodilation, little clinical difference was apparent between devices. With the introduction of corticosteroid medication more thought was required. The aim was to achieve significant deposition of drug in the lung, but to reduce drug landing in the throat and mouth, which contributes to the systemic load with no added clinical effect.

When asthmatic children were first given corticosteroids by jet nebulisation, clinical results were poor. This was predictable because corticosteroids, unlike most other nebulised drugs, are insoluble in the fluids used for nebulisation; they are micronised into small particles and added to a carrier fluid, forming a suspension. Unfortunately the micronised particles of beclomethasone dipropionate in the nebuliser suspension were relatively large. Nebulisation of the suspension generates insoluble drug particles covered by a fluid envelope making them even larger. The baffle system, within the nebulisers used, filtered out the majority of these large corticosteroid containing droplets. This resulted in a very poor drug output and clinical effect. This suspension has been replaced by others which have smaller particles. A greater amount is released from the nebuliser and the clinical effect is better.

Benefits derived by adults from two recent changes in the design of jet nebulisers may not extend to young children. The Sidestream nebuliser has an extra open vent into the nebuliser chamber which causes additional room air to be sucked into the chamber. This extra air pushes many extra droplets out of the nebuliser in a given time. The total amount of drug the patient receives is similar to when using a conventional jet nebuliser but nebulisation time is much shorter. Young children, however, inspire at a lower flow than that generated from the open vent nebuliser. As they will only inhale part of the aerosol laden cloud the amount of drug inhaled may be less than that inhaled from a conventional nebuliser.

The next development (e.g., in the Pari LC Plus & Ventstream) was an additional vent in the nebuliser chamber which is open during inhalation but closes during exhalation. Less drug is lost from the nebuliser during expiration than in the Sidestream. Adult patients can receive twice the dose of drug compared to that inhaled from a conventional jet nebuliser. To gain similar benefit, however, young children must be able to use a mouthpiece or have a complete seal around their face mask. Both are difficult to achieve. Further research is currently needed before these nebulisers can be recommended for young children.

Spacer devices, with face mask attachments for young children, are now the drug delivery device of choice for administering drug aerosols. Several technical issues may have a substantial effect on the dose received:

- Inspiratory valves reduce humidification within the spacer and may improve reproducibility of drug delivery. Resistance of valves has to be sufficiently low for them to open during tidal breathing.
- A large dead space between the inspiratory valve of the spacer and patient may reduce the amount of drug inhaled by young children.
- A high electrostatic charge on the spacer attracts drug containing droplets to deposit into the spacer, reducing the amount of drug available for inhalation. The static charge of a spacer may be reduced by washing it in detergent and letting it drip dry, coating it with an anti-static paint, or making it from a conductive material such as steel.
- Large volume spacer devices deliver considerably more drug than small volume devices. For very small children, however, a small volume spacer may deliver as much as a larger one due to the child's small tidal volume.
- Multiple actuations into a spacer device should be avoided as the pressure effect of the expanding propellant pushes much of the aerosol in the device on to the spacer walls. Drug output is considerably reduced.

Dry powder devices, metered dose inhalers alone or breath-actuated metered dose inhalers are unsuitable for young children because they require greater coordination and less variability of inspiratory flow.

Michael Webb

Dr Michael S.C. Webb, MB ChB, FRCP, is
Consultant Paediatrician and Clinical Director of
Children's Services at Gloucestershire Royal
Hospital, Gloucester.

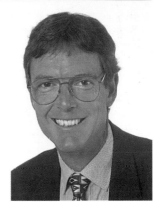

37
What areas should schools' asthma policies encompass?

A school's asthma policy should include guidance on all the requirements
necessary to ensure that every child with asthma receives proper care and
support at school. The policy should, as far as possible, enable regular
attendance at, and full participation in, all school activities. It must be
made readily available to, and understood clearly by, all parents and all
members of staff.

The policy should address the following areas: the legal framework;
individual responsibilities; a description of asthma; a register of children
with asthma; the administering of medication; the management of severe
attacks; education and training; and a list of contacts and addresses.

The law imposes duties on employers to provide for the health and safety
of staff, pupils and visitors at schools, as determined by the "Health and
Safety at Work Act etc 1974" and the "Management of Health and Safety
at Work Regulations 1992". The "Education Act 1993" defines the pro-
visions for a child with special educational needs (which may include special
medical needs). Dealing with medicinal products, including the provision,
storage and administration of asthma medications, is covered by the
"Medicines Act 1968".

The legal responsibilities and accountabilities of individual teaching and
non-teaching staff and parents, within the context of the above acts, must
also be stated in a school's asthma policy. 79

The description of asthma required in a school's asthma policy should include symptoms, common trigger factors, recognition of a severe attack and simple preventive measures. There should also be a description of currently available medications, their mode of action and methods of inhaler administration.

A school also needs clearly defined methods for identifying and keeping a register of all children with asthma, their medications and any other specific information, such as allergies. Detailed individual management plans may need to be kept for some children with severe or complicated asthma.

The method for acquiring and documenting written parental consent for medication to be administered at school must be defined. The policy should identify criteria by which children who can be trusted should be allowed to carry and administer their own medication. It should define which members of staff may, after suitable training, administer medication to children and should set out a system for recording these events and informing parents. There must be a clear plan for the storage and disposal of medications.

A protocol should describe the recognition of acute severe asthma, the treatments that can be initiated at school and by whom, and the steps to be taken if urgent medical attention is required.

The school's policy should state the level of information about asthma that should be incorporated in general education for staff and pupils. There should be specific statements about training requirements for staff who may be expected to supervise or administer asthma medication. An individual doctor or nurse should be named as responsible for providing that training.

Finally, a list of contacts and addresses is needed. This should include emergency telephone numbers of doctors, hospital, etc. It should also contain the addresses and telephone numbers of both local and national support and information groups.

Warren Lenney

Dr Warren Lenney, MD, FRCP, DCH, is
Consultant Respiratory Paediatrician at the City
General Hospital, Stoke-on-Trent, Staffordshire.

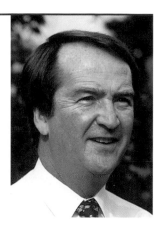

38
Which children should be treated with preventative therapy?

There is ample evidence that in adults with asthma the primary pathology is inflammation of the airways and that inhaled corticosteroids dramatically reduce inflammatory cell numbers, improve lung function and reduce exacerbations. There is less direct evidence in children but it is likely that in most the pathology is similar. Exceptions to this are in the very young—especially in the first two years of life—and in those who only have symptoms associated with mild upper respiratory tract infections, the so-called "viral induced wheezers".

In children with asthma a case can be made for using preventative therapy in a number of situations:

- in very young children before symptoms develop or at the first wheeze in an attempt to prevent the disease from becoming established;
- early in the disease to prevent progression, reduce morbidity and reduce the overall burden;
- in established disease to improve symptoms and lung function, reduce exacerbations and improve quality of life;
- intermittently when symptoms only develop during one season or in certain environmental situations.

At present we have no information on whether preventative therapy in the first two years of life will have any long-term benefits, and the results of studies using varying therapies are eagerly awaited. Many believe that   81 asthma in children is still under-diagnosed and under-treated but that, ironically, in the very young, inhaled corticosteroids are often being over-prescribed in the mistaken belief that they are as effective as in older children. It is also likely that, although prescribed, inhaled corticosteroids are often not given because of difficulties in using inhalers in this age group. Therefore I suggest being very selective in the use of inhaled corticosteroids in this very young age group. If inflammation is inadequately treated, however, permanent damage may occur in the airways and be present in children by the age of six years. Children with symptoms for five years before they commence inhaled corticosteroids show less improvement in lung function than those started on inhaled corticosteroids within two years of developing symptoms. National and international asthma guidelines are all suggesting the earlier use of inhaled corticosteroids in those at risk but we need to identify these children clearly. At present only broad categories are being highlighted, such as those with a strong family history of atopy or a personal history of eczema. These are often not very helpful to the clinician when dealing with an individual patient.

Other preventative therapies, such as cromoglycate, theophylline and antihistamines, which show in vitro anti-inflammatory effects are less effective than inhaled corticosteroids and their use as preventers may hinge on long-term safety issues. Each patient needs individual assessment. When environmental measures and intermittent β_2 agonist therapy are insufficient to keep children well, the early use of inhaled corticosteroids is likely to show most benefit. However, as with the introduction of any other medication, evaluation of that improvement is imperative. When children are asymptomatic it is most unlikely parents will continue to give them regular preventative therapy and to date we have no evidence that inhaled corticosteroids affect the natural history of the disease. Therefore to insist that asymptomatic children continue with preventative therapy is probably impractical and not supported by evidence. Similarly we have no evidence that viral induced wheezing in otherwise healthy children is prevented by inhaled corticosteroids.

In truth, we do not yet know which children should be treated with preventative therapy. However, research studies are beginning to tease out those most at risk of developing long-term disease, and sub-groups of wheezing children will be identified for which there are specific markers (both environmental and genetic) to aid the clinician in individual therapeutic strategies.

Edwina Wooler

Edwina Wooler, SRN, RSCN, NATC Dip in
Asthma Care, is a Paediatric Nurse Specialist at
Royal Alexandra Hospital for Sick Children,
Brighton and the National Asthma Training
Centre Paediatric Course Leader.

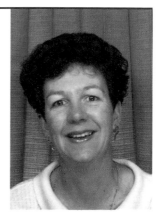

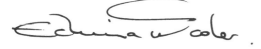

39
How can continuity of care between hospital and general practice in childhood asthma be ensured?

When a child is admitted to hospital with asthma it is a time of emotional upheaval for the child and family alike. The mother, usually the main care giver, has many other logistical headaches to sort out while trying to give her sick child all her attention. The whole family may also be in a state of shock following the child's admission to hospital and may sometimes take very little in at this time. Yet this can be an ideal time to educate the family and to consolidate previous learning as the family members are essentially a captive audience. After the initial crisis management of the acute episode, the nurse should endeavour to discover the level of the family's understanding of asthma. Wherever possible this discussion should also include the child. Many issues of asthma treatment and management can be discussed and an individual plan of care can be reached after negotiation with all parties involved.

Much research has been carried out showing that patients' retention of details is poor and for this reason all information that is given during any consultation should be backed up with written material which is specific to that child. This information is vital once the child is discharged if continuity of care is to be achieved. Not only do the family have mental recall of what has been said but they also hold written evidence to support this. Using this method parents can talk through their management plan with the GP or   83

Practice Nurse during the asthma clinic and any deficit in knowledge can be addressed. It is important that the hospital and practice hold similar views on management and are aware of what each other is saying. Parents easily become confused by conflicting information and may end up "doing their own thing".

Locally agreed guidelines for the treatment and management of asthma are extremely helpful and are being practised in many areas. These guidelines should be agreed by a multi-disciplinary team of health care professionals from primary and secondary health care and should take into account local resources.

Hospitals should ensure that discharge summaries are sent out quickly to the GP so that there is no confusion over medication dosages and plans for follow-up care. Information technology can be utilised to the advantage of health care workers and can also speed up the process of transfer of data by means of fax.

Where a Respiratory Nurse Specialist is employed, it should be a part of the job to ensure that the family have a clear idea about who is going to follow their child up and when. Where this post does not exist, many hospitals have adopted the policy of having a Link Nurse on the ward who will have a similar responsibility. Telephone contact with the surgery when the child is discharged is one obvious way of making contact and discussing the patient's needs. Practice Nurses who have minimal dealings with paediatric asthma patients should find out about local resources so that they can get regular updates in this area. This may involve sitting in on a Consultant Paediatrician's respiratory clinic or a nurse led asthma clinic, or making a visit to the paediatric medical ward to find out about asthma management strategies. Likewise, ward staff should know what each GP practice provides in the way of asthma care. It is vitally important that primary and secondary health care professionals do not work in isolation and that they look beyond the four walls of their ward or practice to offer their patients a complete package of care that is agreed by all.

Chapter 3

Asthma and Related Conditions:
Diagnosis and measurement

David Stableforth

Dr David E. Stableforth, MD, MA BChir, FRCP, is Consultant Physician at Birmingham Heartlands Hospital.

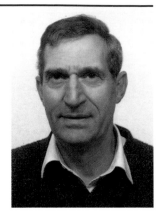

40
Why are people still dying from asthma?

Since the asthma mortality epidemic of the 1960s, asthma death rates in the United Kingdom have plateaued, but total numbers have failed to decline significantly. Asthma mortality still stands at approximately 1600 deaths per annum, of which over half are aged 65 and over. In the 1960s epidemic, patients in their teens and twenties died in excessive numbers and the cause of this is still discussed. Numbers of deaths in young people at that time, however, declined at the same time as non-selective β_2 agonist inhalers were banned from over-the-counter sale. In the 1990s, deaths in young people are if anything declining, particularly in adolescence and childhood.

By contrast, however, there still remains concern about deaths in the elderly, over 65-year-old age group. Here numbers continue to climb. It remains uncertain whether this apparent increase in deaths in the elderly is real or the result of diagnostic transfer or re-flagging. This apparent increase in asthma deaths in the over 65s therefore may be apparent rather than real. Studies are under way to try and discover what proportion of the elderly truly die of asthma.

Confidential asthma mortality enquiries, notably in Norfolk in 1993, have shown that those who do die of asthma often still do so in association with lack of appreciation of severity by patients, relatives and doctors, a lack of monitoring of severity during a patient's lifetime, a lack of oral and inhaled corticosteroid and other prophylactic medication, as well as sometimes less than optimum emergency treatment for severe attacks. Whilst these unsatisfactory features of asthma management were a major problem in the early 1980s, the proportion of patients in whom these factors are important has reduced.

People dying of asthma in the 1990s often seem to be the psycho-socially disadvantaged. These patients often appear to be more socially isolated, may have psychiatric illness, an alcohol habit or just be plain idiosyncratic in their approach to asthma management. Some of them, for whatever reason, are reluctant to visit hospitals and clinics and when they do receive advice they are often non-compliant and fail to turn up to appointments. Some of these patients may hold strong opinions of their own about how their asthma should be managed and prefer not to take medical advice when broncho-spasm is at its worst, often thinking that they can cope on their own.

Prevention of these deaths is going to be difficult. Some clinics have adopted psychological support at special sessions in which patients may be seen by a medical social worker and/or psychologist. It remains to be seen whether this is a useful approach. Certainly a group of brittle asthmatic patients seem to have more psychological problems than patients in a group whose asthma is more stable. It is difficult to know with these patients which is the chicken and which is the egg. Severe and chronic asthma is conceivably likely to make the patients "difficult", but in reality the problem may be that psychological factors are aggravating the asthma.

Some studies have shown excessive asthma deaths in economically poor groups such as the Maoris in New Zealand, but it is less certain whether such factors apply in the United Kingdom.

In order to reduce the number of patients dying of asthma we first need to be sure that our diagnosis is sound, particularly in the elderly. We need to remain vigilant with this group, appreciating that the disease could come on for the first time and behave in a lethal fashion even in patients in their 80s and 90s. Patients with psychiatric illness are always going to be difficult to cope with, as are the lonely and idiosyncratic. The important factor is to realise that this remains one of the at risk groups and to target psychological support to asthma clinics accordingly.

Finally we would need to continue to improve our educational methods for patients so that they can take control of their own disease and also to make sure that everyone who has asthma has access to clinics and specialist advice if necessary.

Richard Harrison

Dr Richard Harrison, MD, FRCP, is Consultant
Physician at North Tees General Hospital,
Stockton-on-Tees.

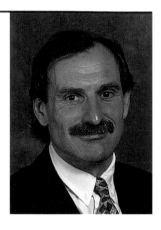

41
What other conditions can be confused with asthma?

Asthma is the only likely diagnosis when a young adult presents with intermittent symptoms of wheeze, breathlessness and cough. Confusion arises when the symptoms are atypical. Breathlessness as the sole symptom occurs in pulmonary embolic disease as well as in the hyperventilation syndrome. Cough as a sole symptom occurs in asthma but it may also be idiopathic ("post viral") and, less commonly, may be caused by post-nasal drip, an inhaled foreign body or oesophageal reflux. Not all young adults with noisy breathing have asthma. The rattle of airway secretions and stridor from upper airway obstruction can both be misinterpreted as wheeze. Excessive secretions may be due to recurrent infection or to a localised area of bronchiectasis. Under these circumstances the sputum will appear purulent and the chest X-ray may be abnormal. Stridor has a harsh superficial quality and is present mainly on inspiration. Episodic stridor, due to unexplained laryngeal spasm, and accompanied by paroxysmal breathlessness is well recognised in young adults, in whom it may mimic brittle asthma.

As the risks for other chest conditions and for heart disease increase, so does the risk of misdiagnosis of asthma. This is seen with increasing age, in smokers, in the obese and in those with important occupational exposure. As symptoms are shared by many of the common respiratory and cardiac conditions, the context in which they occur is all important. The older the   89 patient the greater the possibility that breathlessness and wheeze is due to cardiac failure. Unfortunately, examination findings discriminate poorly between asthma and cardiac failure so if there is a suspicion of heart disease (past history, hypertension or hear murmurs) there is a need for an ECG, a chest X-ray and an echocardiograph. Recurrent aspiration can also mimic asthma and should be suspected in the elderly or frail who present with intermittent episodes of cough, sputum, breathlessness and wheeze.

Smoking increases the risk of chronic obstructive pulmonary disease (COPD) and of lung cancer. Lung cancer can masquerade as asthma. A tumour which obstructs a major airway produces stridor or wheeze accompanied by cough and breathlessness. Symptoms are progressive rather than intermittent and there are often important additional features, most notably haemoptysis, lethargy and local pain. The chest X-ray is almost always abnormal by the time lung cancer produces symptoms.

Interstitial lung disease (sarcoid, fibrosing alveolitis and dust diseases) present with cough, breathlessness and, to a lesser extent, wheeze. Sarcoid has systemic symptoms such as malaise, joint pain and fever which do not occur in asthma. In fibrosing alveolitis the finding of crackles rather than wheeze at the lung bases is an important diagnostic clue. Fibrosing alveolitis is relatively common in elderly patients and in those with collagen-vascular diseases such as rheumatoid arthritis. A history of relevant occupational or recreational exposure will raise the possibility of dust disease. In most cases the chest X-ray provides supporting evidence for a diagnosis of interstitial lung disease.

Philip Ind

Dr Philip W. Ind, MA, FRCP, is Senior Lecturer and Honorary Consultant Physician at the Royal Postgraduate Medical School, Hammersmith Hospital, London.

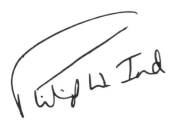

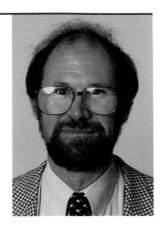

42

What is the difference between asthma and chronic obstructive pulmonary disease?

This is a difficult and controversial area. Asthma is in fact extraordinarily difficult to define scientifically yet most patients and health professionals know what it is. Asthma is a syndrome characterised by *variable* airflow obstruction, bronchial hyper-responsiveness and eosinophilic airway inflammation. Confusion with chronic obstructive pulmonary disease (COPD) arises in several ways.

Firstly, a number of other similar terms are used: COAD (chronic obstructive airways disease), CAL (chronic airflow limitation) and, particularly in the Netherlands, CNSLD (chronic non-specific lung disease).

Secondly, COPD may be used in different ways. The term is best reserved for gradually developing, progressive "irreversible" airflow obstruction related to chronic bronchitis and emphysema—two conditions closely linked with cigarette smoking. Chronic bronchitis is characterised by chronic, persistent or recurrent productive cough (phlegm production each morning for at least three months over two successive years) due to mucous gland hyperplasia in the airways. Emphysema refers to progressive destruction and enlargement of the alveolar air spaces. These two conditions usually co-exist to varying extents in different patients. Unlike asthma, which is defined physiologically, chronic bronchitis relates to symptoms while emphysema is a pathological description (though it can be reliably diagnosed on CT scan). 91

Clinically, asthma and COPD are similar. They often differ only in degree—for example, in the extent of reversibility of airway narrowing in response to bronchodilators (acutely) or trial of corticosteroids (chronically). Some authorities regard the distinction as arbitrary. Mild asthma and typical COPD are readily distinguished by lung function testing etc. However, in many, particularly more advanced cases it may be possible to distinguish the two conditions in an individual patient. This leads to the idea of "overlap" and a patient may be said to have "COPD with some reversibility" or "asthma/bronchitis" or "asthma and COPD". Even more confusingly, a patient during an exacerbation of COPD (with increased variability of airflow and inflammation) may be regarded as "asthmatic" at that time.

Even if the two conditions are regarded as quite separate, they will still occur together quite frequently by chance as both are common. COPD occurs in 15–20% of smokers (who form about 30% of the population in the UK). Asthma occurs in 5–10% of adults. The two conditions will therefore co-exist in about 0.5% of the population.

The vast majority of COPD is related to smoking. However, it is by no means clear which smokers will progress to COPD and why. The idea that an "asthmatic tendency" is responsible for the development of COPD is referred to as the "Dutch hypothesis".

Finally, the term COPD can be used to include other rarer conditions that lead to a similar end result—for example, bronchiectasis, obliterative bronchiolitis, etc.

In summary, there are good scientific reasons for wanting to distinguish asthma from COPD. However, at the present time, the distinction between them is difficult in many patients and is of less importance clinically. Initial management of the two conditions is similar. Therapeutically, inhaled corticosteroids are of proven benefit in asthma while the emphasis is on symptom relief in COPD.

Glenis Scadding

Dr Glenis Scadding, MA, MD, FRCP, is
Consultant Physician in Clinical Immunology,
Allergy and Rhinology at the Royal National
Throat, Nose and Ear Hospital, London.

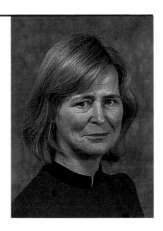

43
How is allergic rhinitis diagnosed and treated?

Allergic rhinitis frequently accompanies asthma and it is therefore useful to
consider the diagnosis and management of this condition in the context of
asthma. The major symptoms of allergic rhinitis are running, itching and
blockage of the nose, and sneezing. Other symptoms may occur, such as
post nasal catarrh, headache, facial pain, reduced smell and taste, and
general tiredness and malaise. These latter symptoms are more common
where the sinuses are also involved.

The diagnosis of allergic rhinitis depends upon taking a careful history,
looking for seasonal and diurnal variation and for any known exacerbating
factors and possible allergens at home and at work. A family history of atopy
or a past history of asthma or eczema make allergic rhinitis more likely. Note
should be made of any medications used, how much and for how long,
together with information on their effectiveness or otherwise. An examination of the patient's nose is carried out, looking for the characteristic
swollen pale nasal lining and any other factors, such as the nature of
secretions present, deviation of the septum, polyps, etc.

Skin prick tests provide helpful supportive evidence of allergens implicated in the patient's history. They are essential when expensive allergen
avoidance measures are contemplated and also provide a useful visual
demonstration for the patient of their allergy. A few test substances, such as
house dust mite, grass pollen, cat dander and feathers, plus a negative

control (saline) and a positive control (histamine), will diagnose the majority of allergic rhinitis patients. Weals 3 mm in diameter greater than the negative control are regarded as positive. Skin prick tests should be avoided in patients with a history of anaphylaxis, or with significant eczema. They may be unreliable in patients with dermographism or in those taking oral antihistamines or corticosteroids. In these cases, blood can be sent for radioallergosorbent testing (RAST), either looking for single specific sensitivities or employing a screen of several likely allergens.

Since allergic sensitisation is initially a local phenomenon it is possible to have a positive nasal response with a negative skin prick test, although this is rare. Such instances can be further investigated by nasal challenge in specialist centres. A simple test is the nasal smear, which can be taken with a cotton bud, smeared on to a slide and examined for eosinophils. These are often present in allergic rhinitis but also in the non-allergic rhinitis with eosinophilia syndrome (NARES); however, both of these respond to intranasal corticosteroids.

As in asthma, allergen avoidance is an important aspect of treatment in allergic rhinitis. Drug treatments for allergic rhinitis depend on the severity of the symptoms. Mild symptoms are treated with antihistamine as required or, if this fails, with local corticosteroids or sodium cromoglycate. Moderate symptoms may be treated (from age four) with local corticosteroids, plus an antihistamine if necessary. In children under four, moderate symptoms may be treated with regular cromoglycate. Severe symptoms are treated with local corticosteroids, together with a short course of oral corticosteroids. In the longer term, sufferers from severe symptoms may benefit from the use of a corticosteroid spray, possibly with the addition of an antihistamine.

A further possible form of treatment for allergic rhinitis is immunotherapy (hyposensitisation). At present the place of such therapy in the treatment of rhinitis is limited to individuals with severe hay fever who are unresponsive to conventional treatment but who do not have asthma. Safer forms of immunotherapy are, however, being sought and may well be more widely employed in the future.

Lawford Hill

Dr Lawford S. Hill, MB ChB, FRCP, is Consultant
Physician at Warwick Hospital.

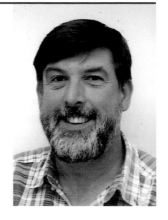

44
How important is the co-existence of asthma and rhinitis?

Asthma is perceived to be an inflammatory condition and rhinitis is simply
inflammation in the nose. Nasal inflammation gives the classical triad of
blockage, sneezing and watery discharge. The majority of asthmatics also
suffer from rhinitis, particularly when allergy is an important factor in
asthma. Rhinitis may be either seasonal (for example, hay fever) or perennial, but is of great importance both because of the secondary effect it has
on the chest and symptomatically in its own right.

The nose is essentially the air conditioner for the lungs. On breathing in,
the air is warmed and humidified. On breathing out, the nose acts as a
condenser retaining water and heat which are then re-used for the next
breath. This lets the lung remain as warm and as moist as possible
throughout the respiratory cycle. When rhinitis is present, mouth breathing
tends to occur, causing drying and heat loss from the lungs. These have
both been shown in experiments to cause bronchospasm in asthmatics and
this mechanism may well be part of the cause of exercise induced asthma.

More importantly, nasal inflammation gives rise to the production of
inflammatory mediators. That these can have a knock-on effect on the lung
is evident from the frequency with which hay fever sufferers can experience
wheezing at the height of the season. This hay fever wheezing can be
abolished by appropriate rhinitis therapy and similarly some asthmatics will
keep their asthma at bay without chest treatment as long as they use a   95

corticosteroid nasal spray regularly. In a group of asthmatic and rhinitic children, the asthma only came under full control once the rhinitis was addressed with an intra-nasal corticosteroid. There were, however, three interesting points which came out of this study. First, that after adding a nasal corticosteroid, asthma control—especially on exercise—was substantially better. Second, that the *inhaled* corticosteroid dose could then be reduced by more than the dose of nasal corticosteroid without loss of control (although it could not be reduced before). Third, that the rhinitis only had to be treated rather than fully suppressed to get these effects.

A properly functioning nose is therefore essential to the proper functioning of the lungs—the nose is after all the upper part of the respiratory tract. In view of this, I regard treating co-existing rhinitis in asthmatics as part of the asthma treatment. Quite often the final step needed to bring an asthmatic to perfect control is to treat their nose just like their lung, using a topical corticosteroid.

Sallie Buck

Sallie Buck, SRN, SCM, NATC Dip in Asthma
Care, is a Practice Nurse in Exeter, Devon and a
National Asthma Training Centre Regional
Trainer.

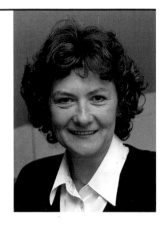

Sallie Buck

45
How strong is the association between eczema and asthma and how can it be managed?

Some adults with asthma also suffer with eczema but the greatest association appears to be in childhood. Both eczema and asthma are manifestations of the atopic condition. Eczema usually presents from 12 weeks of age, with approximately 10% of children being affected by the age of four years. However, point prevalence at four years is 3–4% which indicates that it is already in decline. Asthma generally presents from around three years of age and affects approximately 12–15% of children. Eczema is thus already in retreat by the time asthma is beginning to develop. Many of the children who have atopic eczema go on to develop inhalant allergies. Some unfortunate children have both conditions at the same time, and these will need careful management.

Allergen avoidance in asthma care has been proven to be effective in recent years, with the house dust mite cited as the most important airborne allergen. The house dust mite has, however, only very recently been implicated in the pathogenesis of atopic eczema. Research has shown that reduction of the offending house dust mite and its allergen, by encasing the mattress in mite impermeable covers and regular vacuuming of the carpet, reduces significantly the amount of house dust mite allergen, and has also shown significant clinical improvement in patients with atopic eczema. It is important to stress that allergen avoidance will only be effective in atopic conditions. Therefore in older children and adults it is advisable to prove their atopic status by having a positive skin prick test.

The mainstay of eczema treatment is to keep the skin hydrated and to this end it is recommended that the patient should use regular emollients. However, as with asthma, there is an underlying inflammatory process in eczema and this frequently necessitates the use of topical corticosteroids. These should be used in conjunction with emollients and applied only to the affected areas. Many parents are worried about the use of corticosteroids in their children and frequently under-use them. In asthma management there are guidelines that advise us to start with a high enough dose of inhaled corticosteroid to gain control, and once that control has been achieved to consider reducing the dosage. Similar advice can be given to patients with atopic eczema, with the proviso that once the inflammation has been controlled, the potency of the topical corticosteroid can be reduced and then stopped. Treatment with emollients should continue. Topical corticosteroids can attenuate much of the misery of both asthma and eczema but patients and parents need to have the role of these drugs explained carefully to them, to avoid both over- and under-usage.

Patients suffering from both eczema and asthma may be cared for by dermatologists and also by chest physicians. It is therefore particularly important that the total dose of corticosteroid that these patients receive is properly monitored.

Malcolm Sears

Professor Malcolm R. Sears, MB ChB, FRACP,
FRCPC, is Professor of Medicine at McMaster
University, Hamilton, Ontario, Canada.

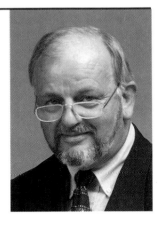

46
What is the relationship between asthma and bronchial hyper-reactivity?

Asthma is characterized by symptoms of breathlessness, wheezing and chest tightness which are generally attributed to narrowing of the airways. The ability of asthmatic airways to narrow excessively has been recognised as the hallmark of asthma. Detection of this ability to narrow excessively and to dilate with treatment have become standard measurements for the diagnosis of asthma. Bronchial hyper-reactivity can be demonstrated by reversibility of airway narrowing, or by showing response to low concentrations of broncho-constrictor substances which do not cause non-asthmatic airways to constrict. Bronchial hyper-reactivity is generally demonstrated by measurements of spirometry before and after serially increasing concentrations of methacholine or histamine. The test is continued until the forced expiratory volume in the first second of expiration (FEV_1) falls by more than 20% from the baseline or post-saline value. The concentration of methacholine which would have induced exactly 20% fall (PC_{20}) is calculated by interpolation on a logarithmic plot of change in FEV_1 versus methacholine concentration.

In clinical studies, virtually all asthmatics with current symptoms show bronchial hyper-reactivity to one or more of the challenge tests performed. However, in epidemiological studies where milder forms of asthma are encountered, not all subjects with symptoms (even relatively recent) show

99

bronchial hyper-reactivity to the challenging substance at the time of testing, while others may have hyper-reactivity without symptoms. In children, up to 30% of the subjects showing bronchial hyper-reactivity defined by usual criteria do not have significant symptoms, while at the other end of the spectrum, about 20% of those with recurrent symptoms of wheezing or with a diagnosis of asthma do not show hyper-reactivity. This has led to some uncertainty as to the usefulness of measurements of bronchial hyper-reactivity in field studies or epidemiologic studies of asthma. To overcome this problem, some investigators have suggested that for epidemiological purposes, current asthma should be defined as symptoms consistent with asthma in the presence of a positive challenge test for bronchial hyper-reactivity. This will detect the great majority of cases of significant asthma but may exclude some with minor symptoms, and also clearly excludes those who have hyper-reactivity without having symptoms.

In general terms, children and adults with clear-cut frequent symptoms of asthma almost always show bronchial hyper-reactivity to a challenge. The less severe the asthma, the less reactive is the airway. Some people with mild asthma that has gone into remission retain hyper-reactive airways while others become non-reactive. Acute viral infections can increase airway reactivity even in people who at other times do not show hyper-reactive airways. Hyper-reactivity is reduced by treatments such as inhaled corticosteroids, and increased by allergic trigger factors in sensitised individuals. There is a relatively good correlation between variability in peak flow rates and measurements of hyper-reactivity.

Freddy Hargreave

Professor Frederick E. Hargreave, MD, FRCP(C),
FRCP, is Professor of Medicine at McMaster
University and at St Joseph's Hospital, Hamilton,
Ontario, Canada.

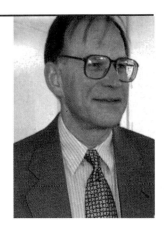

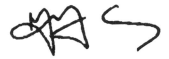

47
How is bronchial inflammation measured and monitored in asthma?

Bronchial inflammation is measured in clinical practice *indirectly* from changes in symptoms, by the need for inhaled short acting β_2 agonist and by means of peak flow (PEF) or spirometry. It can also be measured *indirectly* in hospital practice by changes in airway responsiveness to methacholine (or histamine) or on exercise. It is best measured *directly* by new, reliable and accurate methods of examination of spontaneous or induced sputum cell count. Such direct measurement is, however, currently only available in a few centres in research.

When bronchial inflammation occurs or increases, the various parameters worsen. Symptoms recur or increase and a β_2 agonist is needed more often. PEF monitored on waking at home falls and the diurnal variability (expressed, for example, as highest post-bronchodilator value minus lowest pre-bronchodilator value over the highest value) increases. The PEF or forced expiratory volume in the first second of expiration (FEV_1) or $FEV_1/$ vital capacity (VC) measured in the surgery or clinic falls.

The magnitude of change in the measurements regarded as clinically significant will vary between patients. A worsening of symptoms usually precedes worsening of flow rates. A decrease in flow rates of 10% (measured from predicted value) should be regarded as significant.

When bronchial inflammation decreases, symptoms and flow rates improve. An important objective of treatment is to achieve the least   101 symptoms, the best flow rates and the least variability of PEF. In most patients, the asthma is mild and the best results will be no symptoms and normal flow rates. In some patients, however, some abnormalities will persist in the absence of treatable inflammation, presumably because previous inflammation has resulted in permanent changes in the structure and function of the airways.

It is usual today to consider that an increase in respiratory symptoms in the patient with asthma means an increase in eosinophilic airway inflammation and a need to increase corticosteroid treatment. However, this is not always correct. Recent research with sputum has drawn attention to the different causes and types of inflammation and the different response of these to treatment. The cause may be a specific reaction to inhaled allergens or occupational sensitisers causing an infiltration with eosinophils. Eosinophilic inflammation due to these or other causes tends to respond to corticosteroid treatment. Viral or bacterial infections are more likely to cause neutrophilic inflammation which may not respond to corticosteroid treatment. Therefore, a failure to respond to adequate corticosteroid treatment should alert the doctor or nurse to the possibility that the cause may be corticosteroid resistant and the treatment may need to be changed.

John Rees

Dr John Rees, MD, FRCP, is Consultant
Physician and Senior Lecturer in Medicine at the
United Medical and Dental Schools of Guy's and
St Thomas's Hospitals, London.

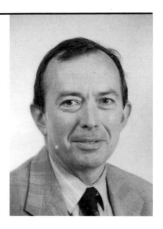

48
What is the place of lung function measurement in the diagnosis of asthma?

Most definitions of asthma include a statement on reversibility of airflow obstruction as a central tenet in the diagnosis. This reversibility is demonstrated objectively by measurement of airflow variations, with time or in response to treatment, and sets respiratory function as a prime investigation in asthma. The common measurements of airflow are the peak expiratory flow (PEF) and forced expiratory volume in the first second of expiration (FEV_1) related to the vital capacity (VC).

In some asthmatics airflow obstruction may not reverse easily with bronchodilators. Consequently, more sustained efforts with bronchodilators and oral corticosteroids might be necessary to demonstrate reversibility. In other patients there may be no airflow obstruction when they are seen between episodes. In these cases, the diagnosis can be established by observing variability of airflow obstruction with time or by challenging the airways to show the increased responsiveness of the asthmatic airway. Challenge can be done simply with exercise or, in certain laboratories, with cold air, histamine or specific allergen. Formal measurement of responsiveness is less common in the UK than in many other countries.

Since peak flow is measured simply on a portable peak flow meter which can be used at home, frequent measurements to assess spontaneous variability can be obtained easily. Diurnal variation averaging 15% or more is a 103 typical finding in asthma. In chronic obstructive pulmonary disease (COPD), FEV_1 and FVC from spirometry tend to be more useful than PEF. The measurements FEV_1 and VC taken from spirometry are more difficult to make at home. In asthma, such measurements add little to the PEF but they may be useful in other causes of airflow obstruction. In localised large airway obstruction, which can mimic the breathlessness and wheeze of asthma, the spirometry trace of volume against time is a straight line showing the fixed flow rate. This is seen more readily on a plot of flow against volume in the flow-volume loop where the addition of inspiratory flow rates provides more information.

In some circumstances more detailed information on peak flow variability is required. This is the case in occupational asthma, where frequent recordings, perhaps every two hours, are needed at work and at home away from any potential exposure.

Other tests can be useful in ruling out alternative diagnoses. Gas transfer for carbon monoxide is a common measurement in many lung function laboratories. The transfer factor per unit of accessible lung volume (diffusion coefficient, KCO) is normal or mildly raised in asthma in contrast to emphysema where low values are typical. Both total lung capacity (TLC) and residual volume (RV) can be measured by helium dilution or by body plethysmography. The RV may be raised, particularly in an acute attack of asthma, but lung volume measurements and airways resistance have little to add in the routine lung function testing for asthma.

Overall, in asthma, the simple tests repeated frequently and accurately are much more valuable than occasional use of more sophisticated tests. The more complicated tests may be helpful in the exclusion of alternative causes of breathlessness.

Jon Miles

Dr Jon Miles, BSc (Hons), MBBS, MRCP, is
Consultant Physician at North Manchester
General Hospital.

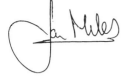

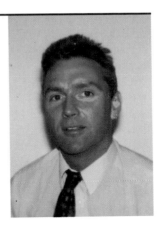

49
What equipment should be used to measure lung function and what are the shortcomings?

Asthma diagnosis is aided by the demonstration of reversible airways obstruction, either spontaneously, or in response to external stimuli such as exercise or an aero-allergen. If an acute attack of asthma is severe enough, the degree of airway narrowing may be sufficient to impair tissue oxygenation. Therefore equipment is required to monitor airway calibre and to measure blood gases.

Airway calibre is monitored using peak expiratory flow (PEF) meters and spirometry. Peak expiratory flow meters are portable, hand-held devices that allow domiciliary measurements of airway calibre to be made to identify the diurnal variation in PEF so characteristic of asthma. The devices are varied but all are easy to use and relatively inexpensive. Their major disadvantages lie in two areas. First, they only provide information about larger airways, whereas asthma inflammation is predominantly the domain of the small airway. Second, in the United Kingdom, their scales are not accurate and this may have implications for both the diagnosis and management of asthma.

It is now common for patients to be issued with instructions to modify their treatment on the basis of PEF changes—the asthma self-management plan—although it is unclear whether all patients with asthma will benefit from this innovation.

105

PEF meters are also available with implanted computer chips which allow accurate recording of the timing of PEF measurement and inhaler use. Patients do not need to write anything down, and healthcare workers can check adherence with greater accuracy.

While PEF provides cheap and easy data on larger airways, measurements of forced expiratory volume in the first second of expiration (FEV_1) and forced vital capacity (FVC) give a greater insight into airway narrowing elsewhere in the bronchial tree. Traditionally such measurements were made on large, dry bellows spirometers, but there are now a variety of portable spirometers available which allow domiciliary measurements of FEV_1 and FVC. Data logging spirometers also exist and are seen by many as the future of asthma self management but at present their expense precludes widespread application.

Flow-volume loops are generated by undertaking a forced expiratory manoeuvre to FVC, followed by a forced inspiratory manoeuvre to maximal inspiratory capacity. Information is obtained about airway flows at all time points up to FVC, and it is this measurement that perhaps best reflects airways obstruction. This information is, however, less reproducible than either PEF or FEV_1. Many spirometers now provide a print-out of the expiratory flow-volume curve. Whether this extra information will be translated into meaningful self-management plans for patients remains at present uncertain.

The determination of arterial blood gas concentrations is an important measurement of lung function in acute severe asthma attacks. Until relatively recently it was only possible to measure arterial oxygen levels by direct sampling of arterial blood. This meant measurement in a hospital setting only. The advent of pulse oximeters, devices capable of estimating oxygen saturation by means of finger or earlobe probes, has meant a potential for oxygen estimations to be undertaken outside hospital. In addition, recent evidence suggests that not all patients admitted to hospital require arterial blood gas estimation either.

Rachel Booker

Rachel Booker, RGN, HV, NATC Dip in Asthma Care, is a Trainer at the National Asthma Training Centre and Leader of the NATC Health Professional's Helpline.

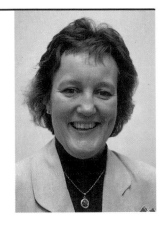

50
How is lung function measured?

Lung function is commonly measured using a peak flow meter or a spirometer. Results are meaningless if the technique is poor.

Predicted peak expiratory flow (PEF) and spirometry values depend on a patient's age. In children they also depend on height and sex. Therefore this information must be accurately recorded. Note also any inhaled or oral drugs that have been taken and at what time. Ideally, patients should not smoke for 24 hours, drink alcohol for four hours, take vigorous exercise for 30 minutes or eat a heavy meal for two hours prior to the test. Clothing should be loose and comfortable. For forced manoeuvres, the patient should have an empty bladder—to avoid accidents and ensure maximum effort! When recording forced manoeuvres, patients are safer sitting upright, well-supported in a chair. Explain the procedure to them and demonstrate it—one demonstration is worth a thousand words. Spirometers must be calibrated and corrected for ambient temperature before each session. Mouthpieces must be clean and preferably disposable.

PEF is recorded on a spirometer or separately using a hand-held peak flow meter. When using a peak flow meter, ensure the pointer is at zero. The patient takes a maximum breath in, places teeth and lips around the mouthpiece, making a tight seal, then exhales in a short, sharp, hard blow, similar to that required to blow out candles. The blow can be discontinued after one second but it needs maximum effort. The highest of three readings

107

is recorded and the pointer returned to zero between blows. The exhaust holes and the pointer must not be obstructed during the test. You should reject blows where the patient has coughed, or air has escaped around the mouthpiece, but do not attempt more than eight blows in a session.

The most commonly recorded spirometric measurements are the relaxed vital capacity (RVC), the forced expiratory volume in the first second of expiration (FEV_1) and the forced vital capacity (FVC). The RVC, where the patient exhales gently from full inspiration to full expiration, should be recorded before the forced manoeuvres. Airway collapse and air trapping may occur with forced manoeuvres and this will make the RVC higher than the FVC.

When recording RVC, FEV_1 and FVC the mouthpiece of the spirometer is used in the same way as that of the hand-held peak flow meter. For FEV_1 the same hard fast blow as for PEF is used. For FVC, instead of stopping after one second, the patient must be encouraged to keep blowing hard until full expiration is reached and he or she is unable to get any more air out. Verbal encouragement is helpful.

A visual display is essential to check that each blow is satisfactory. Reject blows where the patient has coughed, where air has leaked around the mouthpiece, the mouthpiece has been obstructed by the tongue or teeth, where there was a slow start to the blow, or the blow was discontinued before full expiration was reached. Record the highest FEV_1 and FVC from three technically acceptable blows (not more than eight in one session) with a variation of not more than 100 ml.

Some people with asthma develop bronchospasm during forced manoeuvres and consequently the readings become progressively lower. Observe patients carefully and abandon testing if they become exhausted, distressed or develop bronchospasm.

Robert Pearson

Dr Robert Pearson, MSc, MB ChB, MRCP,
D Obst, RCOG, was formerly Medical Tutor at
the National Asthma Training Centre. He lives in
Princes Risborough, Buckinghamshire.

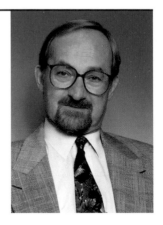

51
What is the place of reversibility testing in the diagnosis of asthma?

One of the important features of asthma is narrowing of the airways, which is usually reversible. The narrowing may occur as the result of varying degrees of the following: contraction of the smooth muscle coat within the walls of the bronchi and bronchioles; oedema within the mucosa and submucosa of the bronchi; and plugging of bronchi with mucus and inflammatory exudate.

Narrowing of the airways is associated with reduced airflow, which can be either detected qualitatively by auscultation (presence or absence of wheeze) or be measured quantitively using lung function tests. The most convenient tests rely upon changes in maximal ("forced") expiratory flow, such as peak expiratory flow (PEF) or forced expiratory volume in the first second of expiration (FEV_1). A "reversibility test" is designed to test for the presence, which confirms the diagnosis of asthma, and the degree and nature of any reversibility of airways narrowing, *at the time of testing*. It should always be borne in mind that asthma is dynamic and changes both during and between days. Lung function may appear to be absolutely normal on one occasion but this should not be taken to exclude the diagnosis of asthma.

There are accepted population-based data for lung function tests, which show mean values with the "normal range", i.e., two standard deviations (SDs) above and below, with allowance made for the age, sex and height of 109 the individual. If the results of the chosen test fall outside the normal range, or there is a suggestive history or clinical evidence of airways narrowing, such as wheezing, a reversibility test may be performed using an inhaled bronchodilator (a short acting β_2 agonist, such as salbutamol, or an anti-cholinergic, such as ipratropium bromide). A positive test, which is an improvement in the chosen parameter of less than 15%, suggests that a significant element of the narrowing of the airways was due to bronchial smooth muscle spasm.

A failure to demonstrate a 15% increase does not necessarily mean that the diagnosis is incorrect or that any reduction in lung function is "irreversible", i.e., unresponsive to treatment. While this might be the case, provided that sufficient bronchodilator was given, then it might be supposed that any residual reduction in airflow attributable to asthma was due to mucosal oedema or "mucus plugging". A "steroid trial" is a reversibility test which gauges the degree of airways narrowing that is due to bronchial mucosal inflammation and which is characterised by mucosal oedema and the plugging of bronchi with mucus and exudate. A positive response to a two week trial of oral corticosteroid is again set at the level of a 15% increase in PEF or FEV_1 and with it the inference that this airways narrowing was inflammatory in nature, making a strong case for inhaled corticosteroid therapy.

This structured approach, combined with a period of home monitoring of PEF, assists the health professional, be they doctor or nurse, to understand the mechanisms within an individual patient. It also helps patients to understand the rationale for their own treatment if the responses are explained to them in simple terms.

Jane Leyshon

Jane Leyshon, RGN, District Nurse Cert, BA (Hons), NATC Dip in Asthma Care, is a Primary Care/Asthma Nurse Specialist with Berkshire Health Authority and a National Asthma Training Centre Regional Trainer.

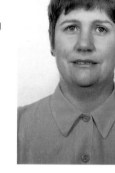

52
How are reversibility tests carried out in the diagnosis of asthma?

The most commonly used medications for diagnostic reversibility testing in general practice are β_2 agonist bronchodilators, e.g., salbutamol or terbutaline. A diagnosis of asthma should not, however, be dismissed if no response is obtained from normal doses of these drugs. Some patients, particularly the elderly and those with concomitant chronic obstructive pulmonary disease (COPD), may only respond to more vigorous therapy and should be tested with high dose β_2 agonist bronchodilators, anticholinergic bronchodilators or oral corticosteroids.

It is recommended that peak flow measurements should be taken near the beginning of a consultation. This allows time, if the peak flow reading is low, to initiate a reversibility test. The waiting time can then be used to complete the history and other investigations. This avoids unnecessary repeat visits and also provides a fuller picture at the initial assessment. If possible, the patient should not take bronchodilator medication in the six hours before the test as this will affect the results. The test procedure is:

- Record baseline peak flow.
- Administer 200–400 mcg of a β_2 agonist, such as salbutamol or terbutaline, via an easy to use delivery device, such as a metered dose inhaler (MDI) plus spacer, or a dry powder device.
- After 15 minutes re-measure peak flow. A rise of 15% or more is significant of a diagnosis of asthma.

- If there is no significant increase in peak flow, proceed, possibly at other appointments, to testing with higher doses (2.5–5 mg). These can be given easily via a nebuliser or by repeated single actuation of an MDI into a spacer device. (Note that in patients in whom a poor response is anticipated, for example in the elderly or those with an element of chronic obstructive pulmonary disease, it might be reasonable to proceed directly to higher doses.)

With anticholinergic agents, bronchodilation takes longer to occur (30–40 minutes). It is therefore preferable to pre-book reversibility tests using these agents and to advise patients accordingly. Where possible, patients should not take bronchodilators in the 6 hours before the test. The longer waiting time during the test allows discussion and may permit other patients to be seen in the interim. The test procedure is as follows:

- Record baseline peak flow.
- Administer ipratropium bromide (up to 250 mcg) via an easy to use device, such as a nebuliser, MDI plus spacer, or dry powder device.
- Wait 30–40 minutes and then re-check peak flow. A 15% rise is significant of a diagnosis of asthma.

A diagnosis of asthma should not be dismissed without assessing the response to oral corticosteroids. The test procedure for this is as follows:

- The patient should record peak flow readings morning and evening at home for a period of one week to establish a baseline.
- Providing there are no contra-indications to oral corticosteroids, prescribe 30–40 mg prednisolone tablets once daily after breakfast. (Enteric coated tablets may be used in cases of known gastric irritation and should be taken prior to breakfast.)
- Ideally, patients should be reviewed within 48 hours of starting the trial and then at weekly intervals to assess for effects and side effects. (Counselling and information with regard to these should be provided prior to commencement.)
- Twice daily recording of peak flow should continue through the trial.
- A corticosteroid trial usually lasts two weeks but occasionally may be extended for a further week if the response is marginal.
- A 15% or more increase in peak flow is significant of asthma. However, some patients may experience improvement in symptoms without a corresponding rise in peak flow, and a more appropriate assessment for them may be exercise tolerance, such as distance walked in 12 minutes before and after a corticosteroid course.
- It is not physiologically necessary to reduce the corticosteroids gradually at the end of the trial, but it may sometimes be desirable to do so for psychological reasons.

Gavin Boyd

Dr Gavin Boyd, BSc (Hons), MD (Hons), FRCP (Edin & Glas) is Honorary Senior Lecturer in Medicine at the University of Glasgow, and Consultant Respiratory Physician at Stobhill NHS Trust, Glasgow.

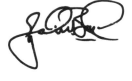

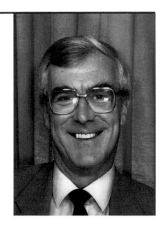

53
What is the role of challenge testing in the diagnosis of asthma?

It is always important to try to establish the causal agent in the diagnosis and assessment of any asthmatic condition. By far the most important approach is to take a detailed and careful history. Further confirmation can then be obtained by performing skin prick tests or by measuring specific immunoglobulin E (IgE) antibodies in the serum. If the causal agent can not be established by these means then challenge by exposure to the suspected allergen would seem to be the next logical step. This, however, is *not* true. Challenge testing, particularly by inhalation, is potentially a very hazardous investigation and should never be considered as a routine investigation. It must be reserved specifically for situations where the identification of the causal agent is of crucial importance to the planning of further management of the asthmatic problem. This basically restricts the use of challenge tests to the area of occupational asthma and also, in certain isolated cases, to the clarification of a diagnosis in suspected food allergy. It is of the greatest importance to understand that allergen inhalation challenges are not without risk and should only be undertaken in specialised centres by staff who have experience in the techniques.

When sensitised individuals are exposed to relevant antigens and an allergic reaction develops, the reaction can be in the form of an acute anaphylactic response occurring immediately after exposure. Major difficulties can, however, also result from the occurrence of severe late asthmatic 113 responses which cannot be predicted and which may not be anticipated with any accuracy from the patient's history. It is also well known that allergen inhalation, not necessarily in high dose, can result in a prolonged increase in bronchial hyper-reactivity which makes the asthma worse and which can persist sometimes for many years.

Challenge tests should, therefore, be reserved only for difficult diagnostic cases of occupational asthma, where the causal agent is in doubt or has not previously or reliably been shown to induce the asthma and, also, where several recognised agents occur in the workplace and the specific agent causing the problem is relevant to decisions about future employment. The use of challenge tests in patients with non-occupational allergic asthma is not recommended and, in the majority of cases, the relevant allergen and the degree of the bronchial reaction can be predicted from a careful and accurately taken clinical history supported by the results of skin tests or allergen specific IgE measurements in the blood.

Sherwood Burge

Dr Sherwood Burge, MSc, MD, FRCP, FFOM, DIH, is Director of the Occupational Lung Disease Unit at Birmingham Heartlands Hospital.

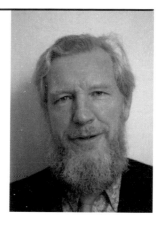

54
How is occupational asthma diagnosed?

About 5% of all adult asthma is caused by work exposures. There should, therefore, be patients identified with occupational asthma on every GP's list. Many, however, may remain unidentified until they are too sick to work, a disaster for the patient. Occupational asthma is particularly important to identify because continuing exposure to trigger factors results in a poorer long-term prognosis. Also, inappropriate advice to leave work can cause severe hardship.

The search for occupational causes of asthma should be included with the search for trigger factors in every adult asthmatic. Patients should be asked whether their asthma improves on days away from work, or on holidays. Those with occupational asthma will usually answer "yes" to one of these questions. Patients with occupational asthma may not be worse when they are at work, as reactions are often delayed for several hours, making symptoms more severe in the evening and night following work. Patients with more than two episodes of sickness from bronchitis in one year should also be screened for occupational asthma, as the diagnosis is most often made in the older smoker, where confusion with chronic obstructive pulmonary disease (COPD) is frequent. Not all those who are better away from work have occupational asthma, however, as improvement on holiday in particular may be due to the avoidance of domestic allergens such as pets.

115

All patients whose symptoms improve away from work warrant further urgent investigation. The British Guidelines on Asthma Management recommend referral to a specialist for all people with suspected occupational asthma. The GP should instigate serial peak flow monitoring as the fist step in the investigation. Peak flow technique should be taught and checked, and performed according to the European guidelines. A minimum of four measurements should be made each day (two-hourly readings are preferable) for at least three weeks. During this period treatment should be kept constant, and times at work clearly marked each day. Analysis is much easier if special recording forms are used. The peak flow records should be analysed by an expert. After three weeks' satisfactory recording, a diagnostic decision can usually be reached. Some people, however, require a more prolonged record to be kept before, during and after a two week break from work.

Peak flow records can confirm the diagnosis of occupational asthma. They can not usually specify the cause. Individuals with occupational asthma should not be advised to leave work unless you think that their disease is so severe that they will never work again. Individuals with occupational asthma should avoid the agent that is causing the trouble. With the patient's permission, this advice should be given to the works' occupational health department, or to the Employment Medical Advisory Service in the absence of an occupational health service. It is then up to the employer to control the exposure, which is likely to prevent further cases.

Joy Conway

Joy Conway, MCSP, MSc, PhD, is Lecturer in Medicine and Physiotherapy at the University of Southampton.

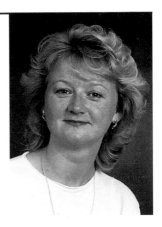

55
What is the place of lung imaging in the diagnosis of asthma?

The diagnosis of asthma is usually made on clinical history. A range of tests—such as evidence of improvement in forced expiratory volume in the first second of expiration (FEV_1) after the inhalation of a bronchodilator; a fall in FEV_1 as a response to exercise; a positive reaction to skin prick testing with a selection of allergens, such as the house dust mite; and increased reactivity to inhaling irritants, such as histamine—can be used to support the diagnosis.

Lung imaging is rarely used to diagnose asthma. It does, however, have a role to play in the acute admission of an asthmatic to hospital, in that a chest X-ray is useful to exclude other reasons for respiratory symptoms, such as a pneumothorax or a lobar pneumonia. It is common to find lung hyper-inflation on an X-ray in an actually ill asthmatic and there may be evidence of small areas of atelectasis as a result of sputum plugging, and these findings are useful clinical information. The more sophisticated forms of lung imaging, such as computed tomography (CT) or magnetic resonance imaging (MRI) scans, would only be used to exclude other diagnoses.

However, there is a more important role for lung imaging in association with asthma. That role lies with the research into the efficiency of the various inhalers used to treat asthma. Drugs or placebo solutions/powders can be labelled with a small amount of radioactivity and their progress into the lungs can be monitored using gamma cameras. Two-dimensional 117 images can be produced that give very useful information on the amount of drug that can reach the lung. It is now also possible to produce three-dimensional images, using a technique called single photon computed tomography (SPECT). In this technique the gamma camera rotates around the body, recording images from many angles, and a computer then recreates the lungs in 3-D. Anatomical information from MRI can also be used to add to the SPECT images. These sophisticated imaging techniques will hopefully give unique information about the site of deposition of drugs and may lead to more accurate targeting of drugs, to maximise clinical effect, in the future.

Chapter 4
Adult Asthma: Treatment and management

Eithne Batt

Dr Eithne Batt, MB, BChir, DCH, DRCOG, MRCGP, is a General Practitioner in Stratford-upon-Avon, Warwickshire and Medical Lecturer at the National Asthma Training Centre.

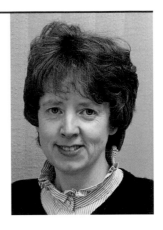

Eithne mßatt

56
How is an acute attack of adult asthma recognised and treated in general practice?

The severity of an attack of acute asthma is often under-estimated by patients, their relatives and their doctors. This is largely because of failure to make objective measurements and can prove fatal. In assessing an attack of acute asthma in an adult it is essential to observe the patient and to make objective measurements of peak expiratory flow rate (PEF), heart rate and respiratory rate. In this way it is possible to distinguish between those with a severe attack and those with life-threatening features.

Features of severe asthma include:
- too wheezy or breathless to complete a sentence in one breath;
- respiratory rate of 25 breaths per minute or above;
- heart rate of 110 beats per minute or above;
- PEF equal to less than 50% of predicted normal or best.

Features of life-threatening asthma include:
- PEF less than 33% of predicted normal or best;
- a silent chest, cyanosis or feeble respiratory effort;
- bradycardia or hypotension;
- exhaustion, confusion or coma.

Patients with severe or life-threatening attacks may not be distressed and may not have all of these abnormalities. Any life-threatening features indicate the need for immediate referral to hospital, although the following 121 immediate treatment should be initiated while awaiting transfer:

- a high dose of inhaled β_2 agonist (salbutamol 5 mg or terbutaline 10 mg), given by nebuliser or by multiple actuations of a metered dose inhaler into a large spacer device (one puff at a time for up to 25 doses);
- a high dose of systemic corticosteroids, either oral prednisolone 30–60 mg or, if the patient is vomiting, intravenous hydrocortisone 200 mg.

The patient should be re-assessed 15–30 minutes after starting treatment and the PEF, heart rate and respiratory rate re-measured and recorded. Any features of a severe attack that persist after initial treatment indicate the need for immediate referral to hospital. Judgement must be used, however, in cases where isolated tachycardia persists, in view of the well-known effects of β_2 agonists on heart rate.

A lower threshold for admission is appropriate in patients:

- seen in the afternoon or evening rather than earlier in the day;
- who have had previous severe attacks, especially if the onset was rapid;
- where there is concern over how seriously they regard their symptoms;
- where there is concern over the social circumstances or the relatives' ability to respond appropriately.

In patients not requiring hospital admission, treatment should continue with a high dose of inhaled β_2 agonist via nebuliser or large volume spacer device every 4 hours, plus oral prednisolone 30–60 mg once daily after breakfast. It is essential that the patient and/or relatives should be given clear verbal and written instructions on how to monitor the patient's asthma at home plus guidance on calling a doctor. For example:

- record PEF before and 15–30 minutes after using the nebuliser;
- call the doctor if PEF is . . . . (give 33% PEF value-predicted or patient's best) or below before using the nebuliser;
- call the doctor if PEF is . . . . (give 50% PEF value-predicted or patient's best) or below after using the nebuliser;
- call the doctor if you need the nebuliser more than every four hours.

In addition, early review should be arranged by the doctor. Oral corticosteroids should be continued at full dosage until PEF has returned to predicted normal or best levels for two days and sputum production has stopped. If the patient was not previously on an inhaled corticosteroid this should be started at least 48 hours before the oral dosage is reduced. If the patient was previously on an inhaled corticosteroid, this will usually be continued during management of the acute attack and then increased to a higher dosage before the oral corticosteroids are reduced.

After recovery it is important to review the circumstances of the acute attack and to educate the patient about future avoidance. All such patients should have a written self-management plan.

Sean Hilton

Professor Sean Hilton, MD, FRCGP, is Professor
of General Practice and Primary Care at St
George's Hospital Medical School, London.

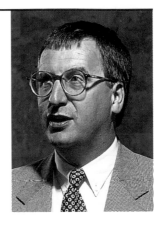

57
What are the criteria for the referral of an asthma patient to hospital?

Referral from primary to secondary care—usually from GP to hospital
specialist in an outpatient setting—lies at the very heart of the structure of
the National Health Service. This "gatekeeper" function of the GP in
directing patients towards the more intensive (and expensive) services
of the secondary sector is seen by most as the key to the relative cost-
effectiveness of the British system of health care. It has been subjected to
increasing scrutiny in recent years. This has revealed wide variations
between GPs in their rates of referral across the spectrum of medical
conditions, including asthma.

Hospital referrals occur for several reasons. Among the more important
of these reasons are: for diagnosis; for management; for reinforcement; and
as a result of patient pressure.

Referral to hospital for diagnosis may be because technical expertise,
usually specialist investigations, is required to make the diagnosis. In asthma
such referral is required if occupational asthma is suspected. Occupational
asthma is a prescribed disease under the industrial injuries scheme, and
specialist diagnostic expertise is desirable. The referral may be because the
referring doctor is genuinely unsure of the diagnosis. This is more likely in
the elderly; in children under two years, where it is increasingly being
accepted that wheezing disorders form a heterogeneous group; and in
adults with persistent unexplained cough.

The referral of a patient to hospital for management may also be for some technical aspect of management which can only be provided in secondary care, or it may be for a complex case beyond the expertise of the person making the referral. Patients with apparently typical asthma who do not respond to high dose inhaled corticosteroids (once adherence, inhaler technique etc. have been checked) would be examples. Infants with asthma also often pose management problems.

Sometimes a doctor will refer an asthma patient to hospital to obtain reinforcement or support for his or her own actions. The doctor may seek a second or expert opinion to ensure that the course of management which he or she is taking is appropriate, but may not wish to hand over management of the case.

In other cases the referral to hospital is made as a result of patient pressure. This may occur because of media coverage of risks of asthma, or may result from the personal beliefs of the patient with asthma (or, more commonly, beliefs within their family).

National guidelines for asthma management have contained sections on appropriate outpatient referrals, and they do emphasise problems of diagnostic uncertainty, or difficulties with management. While this is reasonable, it must be remembered that such guidelines are pragmatic statements rather than criteria based on clear evidence.

Many local factors contribute to the variability in referral rates. Broadly, these are patient factors; general practitioner factors; and secondary care factors. Thus the decision to refer a patient with asthma to a specialist will be influenced by the expectation of, and demands made by, the patient; the knowledge, experience and views of the general practitioner; and the quality and availability of the secondary care services. Because these factors are so variable, the decision about when to refer for specialist opinion must always be an individual one, between practitioner and patient—informed by guideline or practice policy, but not dictated by it.

Brian Harrison

Dr Brian Harrison, MA, MB, FRCP, FCCP, is
Consultant Physician in the Department of
Respiratory Medicine at Norfolk and Norwich
Hospital, Norwich.

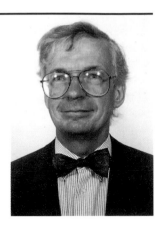

58
How is an adult with acute severe asthma managed in hospital?

Once an adult presents to hospital with acute severe asthma the severity of
the asthma must be assessed. Peak expiratory flow (PEF) is the most direct
measurement of airway calibre. A value 50% or below predicted or best
indicates a severe attack of asthma, and a value below 33% of predicted or
best indicates a life-threatening attack. Remember that patients with severe
or life-threatening attacks of asthma may not be distressed. Oxygen
saturation should be measured and if this is below 92% or if the patient has
any life-threatening features, blood gases should also be measured. Patients
with severe or life-threatening asthma require oxygen, salbutamol 5 mg or
terbutaline 10 mg via an oxygen driven nebuliser, prednisolone 30–60 mg
orally or intravenous hydrocortisone 200 mg or both if the patient is very ill.
Once this treatment hs been initiated a chest X-ray should be carried out. If
life-threatening features are present, ipratropium 0.5 mg is added to the
nebulised β_2 agonist and intravenous bronchodilators are given, either
aminophylline 250 mg over 20 minutes or salbutamol or terbutaline
250 mcg over 10 minutes. Bolus doses of aminophylline should be avoided
in patients already taking oral theophyllines.

If the patient is improving, oxygen, prednisolone 30–60 mg daily or
intravenous hydrocortisone 200 mg six hourly, and nebulised β_2 agonist
four hourly are continued. If there is no improvement 15–30 minutes after
initial treatment, in addition to continued oxygen and corticosteroids orally 125

or intravenously, the nebulised β_2 agonist is increased to every 15 to 30 minutes and ipratropium 0.5 mg added to the nebuliser, repeating this six hourly until the patient improves. If the patient is still not improving, intravenous bronchodilator infusions are started with either aminophylline or salbutamol or terbutaline.

Peak flow should be repeated 15–30 minutes after starting treatment and then measured and charted before and after giving nebulised or inhaled β_2 agonists at least four times daily throughout the hospital admission. Oximetry is also monitored with the aim of maintaining oxygen saturation above 92%. Blood gases should be measured if the patient deteriorates or if the PCO_2 was initially normal or raised.

Patients should be transferred to the Intensive Care Unit if there is a deteriorating peak flow, worsening or persisting hypoxia or hypercapnia, or if there is exhaustion, feeble respiration, confusion, drowsiness, coma or respiratory arrest. Patients do not require intermittent positive pressure ventilation if they are conscious and co-operative and if their PO_2 can be maintained above 8 kPa, or even if the PCO_2 is raised. Ventilation is necessary in virtually all the other situations described above.

As the patient's asthma improves, intravenous bronchodilators and nebulised ipratropium, if used, can be stopped. The frequency of nebulised β_2 agonist can then be reduced from four to six hourly. In the majority of patients, who do not require nebulised treatment at home, nebulised β_2 agonists are replaced by smaller doses inhaled from the patient's usual inhaler device.

Before going home, patients should have been on their discharge medication for 24 hours and had their inhaler technique checked and recorded. Their peak flow should be greater than 75% of predicted or best and the peak flow diurnal variability less than 25%, unless the patient has been seen, and their discharge agreed, by a respiratory physician. Follow-up with their own GP should be arranged within one week of discharge and a follow-up appointment in the respiratory medical clinic at the hospital within four weeks. Patients would usually be discharged on a higher dose of inhaled corticosteroids than the dose they were taking before admission and advised to continue their oral prednisolone until their peak flows reach their usual best levels and remain at those levels for two to three days. Prednisolone can then be stopped abruptly or tailed over six days, depending on the patient's preference. Prednisolone should not be stopped nor reduced if the patient's asthma symptoms remain uncontrolled or their peak flow falls.

Jon Ayres

Professor Jon Ayres, BSc, MD, FRCP, is
Professor of Respiratory Medicine at
Birmingham Heartlands Hospital and at the
University of Warwick.

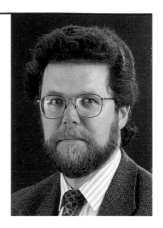

59
What is brittle asthma and how is it treated?

Patients with brittle asthma suffer repeated life-threatening attacks. In type 1 brittle asthma, the attacks occur against a background of widely variable peak flow, despite maximal medical treatment, i.e., at least 1500 mcg of inhaled corticosteroids, regular inhaled bronchodilators and courses of or maintenance doses of oral corticosteroids. In type 2 brittle asthma, repeated life-threatening attacks occur in patients who are apparently well controlled between episodes. Patients with severe "chronic asthma" with persistent symptoms, but who do not suffer life-threatening episodes (i.e., Intensive Care Unit admissions, loss of consciousness or ventilation), do not have brittle asthma.

Type 1 brittle asthma is more common in women (3F:1M). Patients are invariably strongly atopic, usually have significant psycho-social problems and have an increased risk of sleep apnoea. Over 50% have intolerance to at least one food and many have diets deficient in vitamins and minerals. Management is holistic. These are complex patients who need considerable clinical time to address their multiple problems.

Poor adherence to treatment may be present and should be identified, but it should be realised that this cannot explain the underlying severity of their asthma, only an apparent failure to respond to treatment. Dietary causes should be identified on history and, where necessary, by use of a validated food exclusion regime which needs to be undertaken at a   127 recognised centre. Domestic allergen exposure should be minimised—over two thirds of these patients have animals at home but, because they feel that their pets are far more reliable than people, removal is often impossible. "Bartering" to obtain agreement with patients on their management is an important ploy which may have to include suggestions on pet removal. A dedicated psychologist can help both chronic psychopathology and in developing strategies for coping with acutely deteriorating asthma.

Between 50% and 75% of type 1 brittle asthma patients benefit from continuous subcutaneous infusions of β_2 agonist (usually terbutaline), although side effects are significant, particularly at infusion sites. In addition, venous access may be a problem because multiple admissions will have led to permanent loss of peripheral veins. Hickman lines or Vascuports will reduce the unpleasantness of another hospital admission in such patients and may be needed in patients on subcutaneous terbutaline who have painful infusion sites. Corticosteroid side effects are often substantial and may contribute to obstructive sleep apnoea, often of sufficient degree to need continuous positive airway pressure (CPAP) delivered by a nasal mask.

The prognosis for patients with type 1 brittle asthma is variable. Some die, while a few lose their "brittleness", but little is known about the natural history of this condition.

Type 2 brittle asthma is equally common in both sexes. Attacks are characteristically very rapid in onset (often in minutes) and sometimes recovery is equally rapid. Causes are sometimes clear (e.g., peanuts) but are usually occult. It is likely that in most cases an inhaled or ingested allergen is the cause, perhaps resulting in "airway anaphylaxis". Self-injected adrenaline pens (e.g., EpiPen) are mandatory and effective, as are Medic-Alert bracelets (or an equivalent), although patients should be advised, after using adrenaline, to attend the nearest Accident and Emergency Department.

Bill Patterson

Dr Bill Patterson, MB ChB, FRCGP, is Regional Adviser in General Practice for South East Scotland and Honorary Senior Lecturer at the University of Edinburgh.

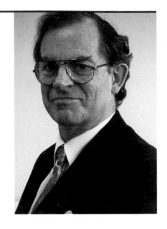

60
Why and how frequently should asthma patients be reviewed?

As prescribers of potent medicines, general practitioners are responsible for checking the effect and side effects of their work. People with asthma often put up with less than ideal control of their condition. They think it is normal for asthmatics not to be able to do things. Good asthma control leads to a normal lifestyle. Pro-active review, particularly of preventer therapy, can transform their world.

The optimum review interval for a particular patient will depend on a variety of factors, such as the stage of diagnosis and treatment, the degree of control achieved and the patient's own wishes. Good, written self-management plans can reduce review frequency. When considering review intervals for asthma patients, the following points may be useful:

- In the diagnostic stage, excess information, too soon, confuses patients. Several appointments at the start can save much emergency time later.
- New patients on the list, or those early in the asthma care cycle, need relatively frequent checking.
- Severe asthma patients need frequent assessment. This can reduce acute attacks. Some brittle asthmatics need direct access facility to a hospital unit for emergency review.
- After nebuliser treatment for an exacerbation, even with good response, review should be within a few hours. Some patients may need to be checked within an hour or two.

- After hospital discharge, review should be within 72 hours. Further plans depend on control levels and compliance.
- The well-controlled asthma patient with no acute attacks may need only annual review.
- Those on high dose corticosteroids may be more vulnerable and need more frequent review. Some practices base the frequency of review on dose levels. The degree of control and absence of exacerbations are perhaps more apt indicators. Very high dose patients need more frequent checks for absorption side effects.
- Some patients/carers can be relied on to use self-management plans safely and effectively. Others need regular doctor or nurse review.
- Some patients will be predictably better or worse depending upon exposure to triggers. Seasonal asthma may only need review in spring and summer.
- With the best will in the world, some patients will not accept advice and will refuse review. Opportunistic checks when they attend for other reasons, and emphasis on a good self-management plan and the recognition of loss of asthma control may help. The patient has to decide in the end.

In conclusion, practices should create their own guidelines of asthma care based on those nationally available. Asthma review may be better done by fully trained Practice Nurses, following agreed protocols. The quality of review benefits from the use of check lists. Asthma patients should have an annual check if they agree. More frequent review will be needed for the various reasons outlined above. A patient's preventer dose should be tailored up or down depending upon asthma control. So, too, should frequency of review.

Duncan Keeley

Dr Duncan Keeley, MA, MRCP, MRCGP, is a
General Practitioner in Thame, Oxfordshire.

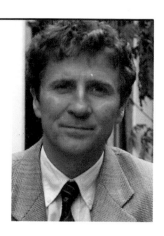

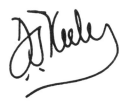

61
What are the benefits and risks of short acting β_2 agonists?

Modern selective short acting β_2 agonists are highly effective bronchodilators. They work mainly by relaxing bronchial smooth muscle, but also
by reducing vascular permeability and increasing mucociliary clearance.
They are best given by the inhaled rather than the oral route because of the
more rapid onset of effect and the much lower doses used. Symptoms of
cough and wheeze are quickly and noticeably relieved, the effect lasting for
up to six hours. We all know about the benefits: what are the risks?

These are extraordinarily safe drugs, though their safety in use in the
treatment of asthma depends on the appropriate concomitant use of anti-
inflammatory agents if symptoms are severe or persistent.

Commonly experienced side effects include fine tremor, nervous tension
(manifested as agitation or over-activity in children), headache and rapid
heartbeat. These effects wear off within half an hour and are not dangerous.
Patients should be taught to recognise them and re-assured that they are
not serious, although the dose or dose frequency might be reduced if
symptoms permit. Hypokalaemia (low serum potassium) may be caused by
high doses, particularly when oral corticosteroids and theophyllines are also
being given. However, acute severe asthma is common and clinically
important adverse events attributable to hypokalaemia in asthma are
extremely rare even in hospitalised patients. It is not normally necessary to
monitor serum potassium in patients being treated at home. Caution is   131

needed when using β_2 agonists in patients with myocardial insufficiency (great risk of arrhythmia) and thyrotoxicosis (worsening of symptoms). β_2 agonists are safe in pregnancy.

What are the risks in an acute attack? Some blue inhalers still carry the legend: "It is dangerous to exceed the recommended dose". This is false. Remember that one 2.5 mg nebule contains as much salbutamol as 25 puffs from a metered dose inhaler, while 5 ml of salbutamol syrup contains the equivalent of 20 puffs. It is actually necessary to exceed the normally recommended dose in exacerbations of asthma if the treatment is to work, provided that medical advice is sought appropriately and treatment with oral or inhaled corticosteroids is initiated or increased at the same time. We inhibit effective self management if we make our patients inappropriately fearful of potential dangers in using their reliever medication effectively.

What are the risks in long-term use? This is more controversial. Some clinicians and epidemiologists believe that regular use of low dose β_2 agonists may make asthma worse in the long run. Others find the evidence advanced for this hypothesis unconvincing. All are agreed that patients who need to use bronchodilators on a daily basis to relieve symptoms should be treated with a regular anti-inflammatory preventer agent as well.

Michael Rudolf

Dr Michael Rudolf, MA, MB, FRCP is Consultant
Physician at Ealing Hospital, London.

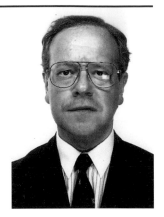

62
What are the benefits and risks of cromones and what is their place in asthma management?

The term cromones refers to sodium cromoglycate (Intal, Cromogen) and nedocromil sodium (Tilade). These are both classified as anti-inflammatory drugs to be inhaled regularly to prevent asthma, but, unlike the inhaled corticosteroids, they are non-steroidal molecules and are therefore totally devoid of all the side effects of inhaled corticosteroids. Their excellent safety and lack of any serious toxicity are their major advantages; nedocromil does have an unpleasant taste, but the Tilade preparation is mint-flavoured to overcome this.

Cromoglycate was first introduced in 1967, and initial clinical trials showed that this drug was an effective treatment in 70% of both adults and children. It was rightly perceived as a major advance in asthma treatment at that time. It is currently indicated for the preventive treatment of asthma which may be due to allergy, exercise, cold air or chemical and occupational irritants.

In adults, cromoglycate's role has largely been overtaken by low dose inhaled corticosteroids, which are regarded as far more effective. Current guidelines still recommend it as an alternative to low dose inhaled corticosteroids in mild asthma; it is certainly worth trying in patients who cannot tolerate (or comply with) inhaled corticosteroids, although nedocromil may now be preferable.

In children, concerns about the possible long-term dangers of inhaled corticosteroids have led to cromoglycate still being recommended as first-line preventive therapy, although many paediatricians and general practitioners do now prefer to use inhaled corticosteroids. Cromoglycate remains both safe and efficacious, although it is rarely effective for wheezing under the age of one year. It is available in dry powder (Spincap), metered dose inhaler (with and without spacer attachments) and nebuliser solution formulations.

Nedocromil is available in a metered dose inhaler formulation. It currently only has a UK product licence for adults and children above the age of 12, although a number of clinical trials have demonstrated its efficacy and safety in younger children as well. It is more potent than cromoglycate, inhibits activation of, and mediator release from, several types of inflammatory cells, and it also inhibits neuronal pathways. New data on its mechanism of action show that it blocks chloride channels involved in cell activation; this may explain its lack of toxicity in comparison to corticosteroids.

Nedocromil is currently recommended as an alternative to inhaled corticosteroids for the prophylactic treatment of mild-to-moderate asthma. A number of clinical trials have shown it to be as effective as 400 µg daily of inhaled beclomethasone. It is particularly effective in controlling asthmatic cough, possibly due to its direct effect on sensory nerve activation. Its only major disadvantage is that it must be taken four times daily.

Nedocromil's place in asthma management is therefore as a totally safe alternative to low dose inhaled corticosteroids in both adults and children. As with cromoglycate, it is certainly worth considering in those patients who may not take inhaled corticosteroids, and it may even be the first-line preventive drug to use in milder forms of asthma where cough is the predominant symptom.

Neil Barnes

Dr Neil Barnes, MBBS, FRCP, is Consultant Physician at the London Chest Hospital & Royal London Hospital (Whitechapel) and Senior Lecturer at St Bartholomew's & Royal London Hospital Medical College.

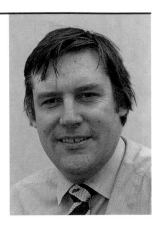

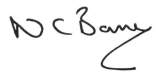

63
What are the benefits and risks of inhaled corticosteroids?

Inhaled corticosteroids are the gold standard controller therapy in asthma. They have a range of benefits not seen with any other anti-asthmatic drug. They improve lung function, decrease symptoms, decrease use of rescue β_2 agonists, protect against antigen induced bronchoconstriction, decrease the number of asthma exacerbations and decrease requirement for chronic use of oral corticosteroids. There is very suggestive evidence of a decreased number of hospital admissions and decreased asthma deaths. There is some evidence, though controversial, that they may prevent long-term decline in lung function in asthma.

In adults at doses of up to 800–1000 µg per day, there is little evidence of any clinically important systemic activity. Above 1000 µg per day in adults, a small percentage of patients will show some suppression of hypothalmic pituitary adrenal axis (HPA axis) function. This percentage rises with increasing doses. In adults this HPA axis suppression does not seem to have any clinical consequences. There is concern though that it may be a marker of unwanted corticosteroid side effects and in adults attention has focused on possible effects on bone metabolism predisposing to osteoporosis. Studies of bone density in patients taking inhaled corticosteroids have shown that they have slightly lower bone density, but much or all of this change may be due to previous courses of oral corticosteroids, poorly controlled asthma causing decreased exercise, which decreases bone mass, 135 and effects of smoking, which also decrease bone mass. The best controlled studies have failed to show any change or have shown a minimal effect of inhaled corticosteroids on bone density. However, this possibility remains the principal worry with high dose inhaled corticosteroids in adults. There is no good evidence of any effect on cataract formation in adults. There are reports of increases in skin bruising and skin thinning but these studies are problematic because of lack of appropriate control groups.

At present a summary of knowledge would be that up to doses of 800–1000 μg per day in adults, there is no evidence of any clinically meaningful side effects for inhaled corticosteroids. Above 1000 μg per day, evidence of systemic activity is present in some patients. The principal worry is that this may cause osteoporosis in some individuals. It is clear that if a patient has asthma of severity that warrants high dose inhaled corticosteroids, then the risk/benefit analysis is in favour of giving high dose inhaled cortico-steroids as the risk of poorly controlled asthma or a requirement for frequent bursts of oral corticosteroids is greater. However, uncritical increasing of the dose of inhaled corticosteroids without clear evidence of benefit is unwise. Many studies are presently being undertaken to better define the long-term side effects of inhaled corticosteroids particularly with respect to bone metabolism.

Anne Tattersfield

Professor A.E. Tattersfield, MD, FRCP, is
Professor of Respiratory Medicine at City
Hospital, Nottingham.

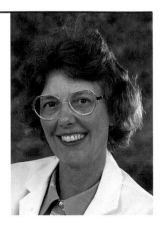

64
What are the benefits and risks of long acting β_2 agonists?

There are two long acting β_2 agonists on the market in the United Kingdom, salmeterol (Serevent) and eformoterol (Foradil). Both are given by
inhalation, both cause bronchodilatation for over 12 hours and both are
licensed for twice daily administration and should not be given more frequently. Both are available as dry powder inhalers and salmeterol is also
available as a metered dose inhaler. The only important clinical difference is
that eformoterol acts more rapidly, achieving near maximum bronchodilatation within 15 minutes whereas salmeterol takes up to an hour. The
rapid onset of action may be seen as helpful to patients although it may
increase the danger of patients taking additional doses to relieve symptoms
if their asthma deteriorates.

The long acting β_2 agonists have consistently shown benefit in longer
term clinical studies compared to placebo, to short acting β_2 agonists
and to theophylline—resulting in a reduction in day-time and nocturnal
symptoms, in improved quality of life and in bronchodilatation that is
maintained over 24 hours. Their efficacy is maintained over several months,
with no evidence of tolerance developing. Most studies have not shown a
reduction in asthma exacerbations, however, perhaps because most were
neither large enough nor long enough to assess this adequately. Alter-
natively, it may be because long acting β_2 agonists do not reduce airway
inflammation (see below).

In terms of possible adverse effects, there have been two theoretical concerns with long acting β_2 agonists. The first is that, like all β_2 agonists, they do not reduce the inflammatory response in the airways. At the end of the day, however, a drug must be assessed by its effect on patients. The second is that by causing prolonged bronchodilatation they may reduce compliance with inhaled corticosteroids. This has only been apparent in occasional patients, possibly because considerable efforts were made to ensure that long acting β_2 agonists were seen as an adjunct to inhaled corticosteroids and not a replacement.

In general, the long acting β_2 agonists have caused few adverse effects. There have been two main problems.

First, acute and occasionally severe bronchoconstriction sometimes follows drug administration, particularly from a metered dose inhaler. This appears to be due to the excipient in the inhaler rather than the β_2 agonist. It probably occurs more often with salmeterol, presumably because of its slower onset of action. Long acting β_2 agonists should not therefore be given during episodes of deteriorating asthma.

Second, there are the adverse effects that are seen with all β_2 agonists—palpitations, headache, tremor, cramps and a fall in serum potassium. The main difference is that with long acting β_2 agonists these are likely to last longer. Such effects are rare with recommended doses of salmeterol and eformoterol but the therapeutic window is relatively small and occasional patients have adverse effects with recommended doses.

In conclusion, the long acting β_2 agonists are more efficacious than placebo, than regular short acting β_2 agonists or than theophylline. Their main adverse effects are occasional bronchoconstriction and systemic effects which may include palpitations, tremor, headache and hypokalaemia. Adverse effects are relatively uncommon when the drugs are given twice daily only and in recommended dose.

Andrew Greening

Dr Andrew P. Greening, BSc, MB ChB, FRCPE, is
Consultant Physician at Western General
Hospital NHS Trust, Edinburgh and Part-time
Senior Lecturer at the University of Edinburgh.

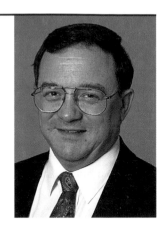

65
When should a long acting β_2 agonist be introduced rather than the dosage of inhaled corticosteroids increased?

The question is carefully phrased. Long acting β_2 agonists should not be used alone, instead of inhaled corticosteroids, but should be added to an existing regimen of inhaled corticosteroid. There are three principal circumstances where such a strategy may be useful: first, for specific control of nocturnal symptoms; second, for long duration control of exercise-induced asthma; and third, for improvement in lung function and control of symptoms in patients who have regular symptoms but whose asthma, generally, is not unstable (i.e., they are not experiencing frequent exacerbations).

Symptoms during the night and first thing on awakening are common and may well occur when the patient has no or minimal day-time symptoms. Long acting β_2 agonists have been shown in many studies to reduce nocturnal awakening and to reduce the overnight fall in lung function, and they have been more effective and have had fewer unwanted effects than alternative agents. Inhaled corticosteroids alone may resolve nocturnal asthma, but by no means always. There are no studies to determine the precise dose of inhaled corticosteroid at which the addition of a long acting β_2 agonist may be more effective than simply increasing the corticosteroid dose, but $800 \, \mu g/day$ (as for poorly controlled symptoms, see below) appears a reasonable estimate.

139

β_2 agonists are very effective in preventing exercise-induced symptoms. The long acting β_2 agonists may provide similar protection for a longer time. In the largest study in teenagers and young adults (more than 160 patients) complete protection was seen with salmeterol and with salbutamol on immediate exercise challenge in about 80% of patients. The long acting β_2 agonist still provided complete protection $11\frac{1}{2}$ hours after dosing for about 60% of patients. School children, with their wide range of spontaneous exercise, and at some schools less than immediate access to their inhaler, may seem the most likely beneficiaries of this use of a long acting β_2 agonist.

Turning now to the treatment of symptomatic asthma, two large studies—one UK-based in general practice and the other international-based in hospital practice—have shown that adding a long acting β_2 agonist to the existing dose of inhaled corticosteroid is more effective than doubling the dose of inhaled corticosteroid in terms of improving lung function and symptom control. The former study, which looked at a starting dose of inhaled corticosteroid of 400 μg/day, was less impressive with respect to the symptom control than the latter, which had a starting dose of inhaled corticosteroid of 800-1000 μg/day. In another study, double-blind crossover against placebo in design, the addition of a long acting β_2 agonist allowed improved lung function and improved symptom control while the dose of inhaled corticosteroid was adjusted downwards (677 μg/day with placebo, 563 μg/day with the long acting β_2 agonist). These data suggest that when the daily dose of inhaled corticosteroid is about 800 μg the addition of a long acting β_2 agonist may be a better alternative to increasing the dose of inhaled corticosteroid for control of symptoms.

Let me end with a word of caution. All patients are individuals and not simply the mean of a large number. Some will not benefit from the use of a long acting β_2 agonist. When therapy is changed we must observe each patient to determine that the desired benefit has been achieved.

Clive Page

Professor Clive P. Page, BSc, PhD, is Professor
of Pharmacology at King's College, University of
London, and Co-Director of the Sackler Institute
of Pulmonary Pharmacology, King's College
Hospital Medical School, London.

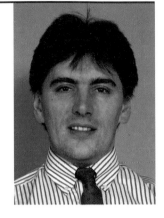

66
What are the befits and risks of theophyllines and what is their place in asthma management?

Theophylline has been used in the treatment of asthma since the turn of the century. It has been widely used as a bronchodilator, both for the management of chronic asthma and the treatment of acute severe asthma. However, since the introduction of inhaled β_2 agonists and inhaled glucocorticosteroids, theophylline has been used less and less, largely because the therapeutic window is very narrow (5–15 $\mu g/ml^{-1}$, and adverse effects are associated with plasma levels above 20 $\mu g/ml$).

Recent data have suggested that theophylline may possess other actions than bronchodilatation at lower plasma levels leading to a re-appraisal of this drug. Thus, theophylline (200 mg twice daily) has been shown to possess anti-inflammatory activity. Theophylline has been reported to reduce allergen-induced eosinophil infiltration into the airways of asthmatics, assessed by biopsy, and to alter the function and activity of T-lymphocytes in asthmatics. Furthermore, in placebo controlled studies, withdrawal of theophylline from corticosteroid-dependent asthmatics has been shown to lead to worsening of asthma and to worsening of the inflammatory cell profile of biopsies obtained from these asthmatics. These data support the concept that theophylline has important anti-inflammatory and immuno-modulatory activities clinically that may be complementary to corticosteroids.

The current British Guidelines on Asthma Management for the treatment of chronic asthma put theophylline as an add-on therapy if control is not gained with β_2 agonists and corticosteroids. However, the recent WHO guidelines Committee has placed theophylline at level 2 and suggest that this drug should be considered as an alternative to cromolyn in children or to low dose inhaled corticosteroids. Clearly, low dose theophylline has a better safety profile than the higher doses required to achieve bronchodilatation. Given the increased compliance associated with oral medications, such as theophylline, and the fact that it is one of the cheapest medications available, it would seem timely to consider the wider use of low dose theophylline in the management of mild to moderate asthma.

Tim Clark

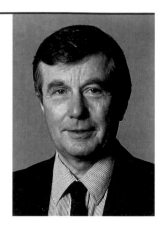

Professor T.J.H. Clark, MD, BSc, FRCP, is Dean and Professor of Pulmonary Medicine at the National Heart and Lung Institute, Imperial College of Science, Technology and Medicine, London and Consultant Physician at the Royal Brompton Hospital, London.

67
What are the benefits and risks of oral corticosteroids?

Corticosteroids are used to treat asthma in two ways. Firstly, they are used for acute severe asthma, when they are frequently given by intravenous infusion. Secondly, they are used for chronic asthma when it is severe and unresponsive to other treatment.

The effectiveness of corticosteroids in acute severe asthma has been queried but they remain standard treatment, often being given orally since the advantage of intravenous treatment is debatable. As treatment is brief and intensive, even in high doses given orally, side effects are unusual. Change in mood is occasionally troublesome and control of diabetes may be more difficult. Brief treatment with oral corticosteroids for acute severe asthma is thus generally recommended, with probable benefit preferred to the risk of asthma fatality and short-term side effects of therapy.

Oral corticosteroids, by contrast, are undoubtedly effective in the majority of patients with chronic asthma who have exacerbations. It is necessary to distinguish exacerbations from asthmatic episodes (which respond well to inhaled β_2 agonists). Exacerbations are associated with a progressive worsening of symptoms, which are unresponsive to broncho-dilators and which, when acute and severe, can be life-threatening. As discussed above, these require treatment with a short, high dose course of corticosteroids. Inhaled corticosteroids are particularly effective in reducing the rates of less acute and less severe exacerbations, and have reduced the

143

use of oral corticosteroids very considerably, while improving control of asthma and quality of life. This is fortunate since oral corticosteroid treatment frequently carries with it unwanted systemic side effects when used regularly for chronic asthma.

Occasional short courses of oral corticosteroids can thus be safely used to treat either acute severe asthma or exacerbations of chronic asthma, despite causing a temporary perturbation of the hypothalamus pituitary adrenal (HPA) axis. By contrast, chronic treatment with oral corticosteroids suppresses adrenal function and has a wide variety of unwanted side effects, some of which can be severe. In particular, oral corticosteroids may cause osteoporosis in adults and stunting of growth in children.

As a result, oral corticosteroids are reserved for short-term treatment of exacerbations which are uncontrolled by inhaled corticosteroids and bronchodilators. Occasionally, however, this conventional therapy is unable to prevent recurrent exacerbations, and chronic dosing with oral corticosteroids is required. Inhaled corticosteroids can be used in high doses to minimise the oral dose and its side effects, and some authorities also recommend oral corticosteroid treatment on alternate days to minimise adverse side effects.

In summary, as a general rule, oral corticosteroids should be reserved primarily for short course treatment of exacerbations and, in the lowest dose possible, for maintenance therapy when conventional treatment can neither control exacerbations nor sufficiently improve quality of life.

Paul O'Byrne

Professor Paul O'Byrne, MB, FRCPI, FRCP(C), is
Professor of Medicine, McMaster University,
Hamilton, Ontario, Canada.

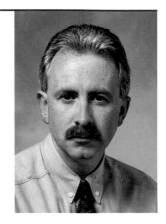

68
What is the ideal oral corticosteroid dosage regime for adults?

Glucocorticosteroids have been used to treat a variety of airway diseases
since the early 1950s. Cortisone was the first corticosteroid developed for
clinical application. Before the end of the 1950s, hydrocortisone, prednisolone, methylprednisolone, prednisone, triamcinolone and dexa-
methasone had been developed and were in clinical use. Cortisone and
prednisone are pro-drugs, which require hydroxylation in the liver to the
active compounds hydrocortisone and prednisolone.

Current practice reserves the systemic administration of corticosteroids in
asthma for patients with acute severe asthma, or for patients with severe
asthma who remain symptomatic despite the use of other conventional
treatments, or to establish what is optimal asthma control in newly evaluated patients.

Corticosteroids, such as prednisone or methylprednisolone, are rapidly
and completely absorbed across the gastro-intestinal tract and have a very
high oral bio-availability. Therefore, intravenous glucocorticosteroiods
need only be used to treat airway diseases in exceptional circumstances, such
as patients who cannot swallow, or who are vomiting. Despite this, intravenous methylprednisolone (for example, 125 mg intravenously three times
daily) is recommended by most consensus documents on the treatment of
acute severe asthma. Most severe asthma exacerbations, however, can be
adequately treated with oral prednisone or prednisolone (0.5–1 mg/kg/

145

day, or its equivalent).This can be administered as a once daily dose. Oral corticosteroids should be started in all patients considered to have acute severe asthma, as indicated by an increase in symptoms (day-time and/or nocturnal), an increase in β_2 agonist use for symptom relief over the past 24–48 hours, and airflow obstruction, as indicated by a reduction in peak flow (PEF) or forced expiratory volume in the first second of expiration (FEV_1) from best value. They should be continued until patients have fully recovered and have regained optimal asthma control. This is usually five to seven days of treatment, but can be as long as 14 to 21 days. The oral corticosteroids should never be stopped until the patient has been evaluated by the healthcare professional managing their asthma. In patients who are using oral corticosteroids infrequently (once or twice each year), the medication can be stopped without tapering the dose. In patients who are using oral corticosteroids more frequently, the medication should be tapered over five to seven days to minimise withdrawal effects.

In patients with chronic poorly controlled asthma, regular use of oral corticosteroids may be needed to attempt to achieve optimal control. The dose used should be reduced to the minimal needed to maintain control, and ideally should be administered on alternate days, to reduce the risk of unwanted effects.

In asthmatic patients being newly assessed, a trial of oral corticosteroids is often used to establish the patient's optimal asthma control and best values of lung function. Similar doses of corticosteroids are used to those used for acute severe asthma, i.e., 0.5–1 mg/kg/day of prednisolone administered once daily for three to four weeks of treatment. Once optimal asthma control is established, the oral corticosteroids are replaced by other anti-asthma medications, most usually inhaled corticosteroids, to maintain control.

Dermot Ryan

Dr Dermot P. Ryan, MBBChB, MRCGP,
DObstRCOG, is a General Practitioner in
Loughborough, Leicestershire. He is Chairman of
the GPs in Asthma Group.

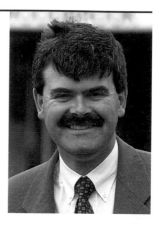

69
What are the issues surrounding nebuliser use in general practice?

Nebulisers have become an everyday tool in the management of respiratory disease in general practice. Nearly every practice possesses at least one, and the majority of general practitioners carry one in the boot of their car for emergencies. There has also been a tremendous growth in the use of nebulisers at home, and many of our patients see them as the gold standard of respiratory care.

There is little doubt that for some of our patients, especially those with chronic obstructive pulmonary disease and cystic fibrosis, nebuliser systems have become essential devices for treatment administration. Equally they have proved their worth in the acute situation, particularly when the patient is panicking or is otherwise unable to follow instructions, making the use of multiple actuations of a β_2 agonist through a large volume spacer impossible.

However, although use of nebuliser systems is commonplace as a means of treatment administration, nebulisers have not been subject to rigorous scientific assessment or evaluation; small scale studies suggest a need for urgent review and rationalisation of current practice. The long awaited British Thoracic Society guidelines on nebuliser use should act as a springboard for change.

The work that has been done suggests that a number of areas would be suitable for improvement:

- Check with the manufacturer that nebulisers and compressors are compatible. It is important that the compressor generates an adequate flow of compressed air to nebulise the solution containing the medication.
- Find out if any local management plans have been developed, and determine who is responsible for your local nebuliser therapy services.
- Give patients written self-management plans, so that they are not confused about which medication to use and when to use it, and when and where to seek advice during exacerbations.
- Ensure consistency of advice about filling the nebuliser chamber, and the time needed to nebulise a given solution.
- Ensure that the patient has information about maintaining and cleaning the nebuliser/compressor combinations.
- Ensure that the patient has information about consumables, for example tubing and masks, and how replacements can be obtained.
- Review of patient's therapy regularly.

As already mentioned, many patients attach undue value to nebulisers and hold them in very high regard. These views need to be moderated by a package of education tailored to the needs of the individual patient. It is important that the most suitable system is chosen, for example pressurised metered dose inhaler plus spacer device or dry powder device may be the most appropriate, ensuring undue psychological reliance is not placed on a machine. As practitioners, we need to be alert to those patients who fail to seek medical advice in a deteriorating situation because of over-reliance on their home nebuliser system.

Consideration also needs to be given to the costs involved. The capital outlay on the average good quality electric nebuliser is about £120. In addition there is the much smaller cost of the nebuliser chamber and consumables. These costs pale into insignificance compared to the costs of the medications. For example, the cost of a patient on 500 mcg budesonide twice daily and 2.5 mg salbutamol once daily would be around £1400 a year using the most efficient systems.

It is desirable that each health authority has its own guidelines on the use of nebuliser systems to enable a consistent approach in their utilisation. Such a strategy would include a centralised point for the distribution, maintenance and repair of compressors; it could act as a resource for queries concerning all aspects of nebulised therapy. This service should be able to provide patients with replacement systems at short notice in case of mechanical failure.

In summary, nebuliser systems will be with us for a long time yet. They are invaluable for selected patients, but as therapists we need to improve our standards of practice to optimise the use of nebulised medications.

Steve Newman

Dr Steve Newman, PhD, F Inst P, FIPEMB, is
Research Director at Pharmaceutical Profiles Ltd,
Nottingham.

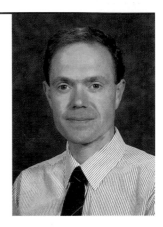

Steve Newman

70
What is the ideal way to use and maintain a spacer device?

Several types of spacer device are available as attachments to pressurised
metered dose inhalers (pMDIs). Most of these devices are large "holding
chambers" such as the Nebuhaler, Volumatic and Fisonair, with a one-way
valve in the mouthpiece, and this answer will concentrate on the use of
devices with this design.

Patients should fire a dose into the spacer and start to inhale immediately.
It is possible for the MDI spray to be fired into the spacer and "stored"
there momentarily before inhalation commences, but the delay time
between firing and inhaling should be as short as possible. Delay times
longer than one or two seconds may result in a significant "rain out" of
particles on to the spacer walls, with a resulting loss in the delivered dose.

Ideally, the patient should take a slow deep inhalation from the spacer,
and follow this with 10 seconds breath holding. However, relaxed tidal
breathing of a single dose from the spacer is an acceptable alternative, and
may be the most practical inhalation technique, especially in children.

The MDI should only be fired into the spacer once before inhalation
starts. If the MDI is fired more than once, then the losses on the walls
increase, and the spacer does not deliver drug as efficiently as with a single
firing. When large doses involving many puffs are required, it may be
considered convenient to fire a number of doses into the spacer and to ask
the patient to inhale them all in one go, or to fire doses into the spacer as the

patient breathes tidally. However, it should be borne in mind that the efficiency of the spacer using these methods will be reduced compared with that achievable by inhaling single doses.

Most spacer devices are made of plastic, and acquire a static charge. This results in drug particles being attracted to the spacer walls, so that they are no longer available for the patient to inhale. New spacers taken straight out of their wrappings may be highly charged, and hence may be relatively inefficient in delivery drug. Recent work from our laboratory suggests that washing spacers prior to use in soapy water, rinsing in clean water and allowing the spacer to dry has a "priming" effect that reduces static charge, and which consequently increases the drug dose that the patient receives. However, the problems of static charge build-up are complex, and the consequences for drug delivery are incompletely understood at the present time.

Graham Crompton

Dr Graham K. Crompton, MB ChB, FRCPE, FCCP, is Consultant Physician at the Respiratory Unit, Western General Hospital, Edinburgh and Senior Lecturer in the Department of Medicine at the University of Edinburgh.

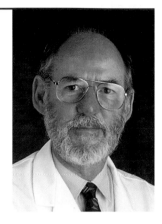

71
Which are the most recent delivery systems available and what are their advantages and disadvantages?

The conventional pressurised metered dose inhaler (pMDI), which is now over 40 years old, was improved greatly when it was made breath-actuated (Autohaler), since this overcame the need for co-ordinating dose release with inspiration, which is found difficult by a large number of patients. The Easi-Breathe breath-actuated pMDI is a better device than the Autohaler, because it is triggered at a slightly lower inspirational flow and it has an in-built resistance. The resistance to air flow through the device makes patients breathe in slowly after the dose has been released, which is the most efficient way of inhaling drug from a pMDI.

Breath-actuated devices do not overcome the problem that a substantial minority of patients have of not being able to continue breathing in once the pMDI propellants have been released into the mouth and pharynx (cold-Freon effect). The spacehaler is a modified pMDI which slows down the speed at which the aerosol cloud is ejected from the mouthpiece of the inhaler. This is achieved by converting the linear aerosol jet into a slowly moving vortex, which also has the advantage of allowing large particles in the aerosol cloud to be deposited in the inhaler mouthpiece and thus decreasing oropharyngeal deposition. The Spacehaler may also increase lung deposition of drug, and, therefore, has many of the advantages of holding chambers such as the Nebuhaler, Volumatic and Aerochamber, but 151 it is much smaller than these large volume spacers. The Spacehaler is, however, more bulky than the conventional pMDI.

Dry powder inhalers (DPIs) have many advantages over the pMDI, but unfortunately they are all more expensive. Single dose DPIs are, in general, less costly than multi-dose devices, but are not as popular with most patients. The Turbohaler is undoubtedly a popular and commercially successful device and refinements to it and new inhalers using the gravity feed system will soon be available.

The minute amount of drug particles delivered from devices like the Turbohaler can be a problem with some patients, since they do not get any sensation that any drug has been inhaled. This is not a problem with most new patients who have not used any kind of inhaler before, but can lead to concern in those who are changed from a pMDI to a "drug only" DPI, since they are used to the propellant—which many believe is the drug—being delivered into their mouths.

DPIs which use drug mixed with a carrier powder such as lactose (most if not all single dose devices such as the Rotahaler) provide patients with the sensation of inhaling their drug but the relatively large amounts of carrier powder in these drug capsules/cartridges and in the "blisters" of the Diskhaler Disks are found to be unpleasant by some patients and sometimes can cause cough. Cough is much more troublesome, however, with pMDI inhalers, mainly because of the surfactants/lubricants which they have to contain to ensure repeated accurate valve functioning.

The 60 dose Accuhaler, which uses a "foil strip blister system" and a small quantity of lactose carrier, is a much better device than any other currently available delivery system which uses the principle design feature of "each dose being individually packaged". The dose counter on this device is also a welcome feature.

Unfortunately, all the recent advances in delivery systems have made inhalation therapy more simple only for adults. Children under the age of about five have been somewhat neglected!

Peter Barnes

Professor Peter Barnes, DM, DSc, FRCP, is
Professor of Thoracic Medicine at the National
Heart and Lung Institute, Imperial College of
Science, Technology and Medicine, London, and
Consultant Physician at the Royal Brompton
Hospital, London.

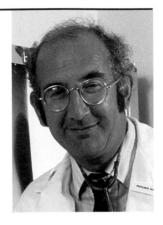

72
What are the new drugs for asthma and what are their mechanisms?

It has proved difficult to develop new classes of drug for the treatment of
asthma despite considerable effort on the part of the pharmaceutical
industry. This is because currently used therapies are so safe and effective.
Inhaled β_2 agonists are by far the most useful bronchodilators available and
inhaled glucocorticoids are the most effective anti-inflammatory treatment.
In combination they will control most asthmatic patients if used correctly.
New drugs recently introduced into the asthma market are improvements
on existing classes of drug and include long-acting inhaled β_2 agonists
(salmeterol and formoterol) and a new inhaled glucocorticosteroid (fluticasone propionate).

Anti-leukotrienes are the only new class of anti-asthma drug to reach the
market in the last 20 years. These drugs include leukotriene receptor
antagonists and inhibitors of the enzyme 5-lipoxygenase which is key to
their synthesis (and both types of inhibitor seem to have a similar clinical
effect). Leukotrienes are inflammatory mediators that are abnormally produced in asthma and can cause bronchoconstriction, plasma exudation and
mucus secretion. Anti-leukotrienes reduce allergen-, exercise-and cold air
induced asthma (by 40–70%) and completely block aspirin-induced asthma
in aspirin-sensitive asthmatics. In clinical trials these drugs improve lung
function, reduce symptoms and reduce the need for bronchodilator rescue
therapy. Their great advantages are their apparent lack of class-specific side

153

effects (so far) and their effectiveness when given by mouth. However, as expected, they are less effective than inhaled corticosteroids. It is possible that some types of asthma patient (such as aspirin-sensitive patients) may respond better than others and when these drugs become widely available it may be possible to select patients or to give a trial of therapy.

Many new drugs are currently in development for asthma therapy. These include phosphodiesterase 4 inhibitors, which are both bronchodilator and anti-inflammatory, but which are currently causing problems with side effects, such as nausea and headaches. Other new drugs include antibodies to immunoglobulin E (IgE), to prevent triggering of the allergic response with allergen; antibodies to interleukin-5, to prevent eosinophil inflammation; and immunomodulators, which interfere with the immune mechanisms underlying the inflammatory response. These latter drugs would also be effective in other allergic diseases. It would be nice to find a once-a-day tablet that would control asthma without any side effects, or preferably a cure! This may be possible when much more is understood about the molecular switches involved in the causation of asthma.

John Hall

Dr John R. Hall, MB ChB, FFPM, DRCOG, DIH,
AFOM, is Chief Executive of Dr John Hall &
Associates Ltd, Dogmersfield, Hampshire.

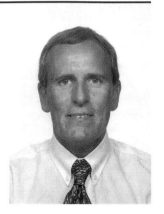

73
Are the generic inhalers bio-equivalent to branded products?

Generic inhalers *are* equivalent to branded products because they have been
licensed by the Medicines Control Agency on the basis of being "essentially
similar". Nothing is quite that simple, however, and I will address the issues
in more detail.

Drugs developed for use by the inhaled route undergo a battery of in-
vitro and in-vivo tests. It is important to test in-vitro for consistency of dose
delivered and particle size distribution (a major determinant of whether the
drug reaches the periphery of the lung or not). More important than in-
vitro testing, however, is the need for clinical data. The ease of acquiring
data in patients depends upon whether we are dealing with a reliever
(bronchodilator) or a preventer medicine. Bronchodilators are far easier to
test, since a single dose will give an improvement in lung function, which
can be compared with the effect of the branded alternative. It is far more
difficult to test preventer drugs, however, since the response is gradual and
takes effect over a period of days or weeks. Furthermore, the scope for
performing pharmaco-kinetic tests (to discover how the drug is handled by
the body) is very limited with inhaled drugs. The amount of drug inhaled is
so small that the level in the blood is barely measurable.

Given these difficulties, it is vital to perform adequate tests of therapeutic
efficacy and safety to establish clinical equivalence. This is best achieved by
testing the generic inhaler in comparison with the branded one in various 155

patient groups (children, adults and the elderly) and in patients with varying degrees of asthma severity. Again, this is relatively easy with reliever medicines in single-dose or short-term experiments, but needs extended research (studies lasting at least four weeks) to confirm the equivalence of preventer medicines. Such research is expensive and may deter many generics companies from entering into competition, or may persuade them to rely on in-vitro data only.

Until relatively recently in the UK and the USA it was possible to license generic inhalers largely on the basis of in-vitro equivalence only. Recent changes in licensing attitudes, however, now call for clinical evidence of equivalence rather than simply comparing their physical performance. Even this raises difficulties because of the disease area itself. Asthma is such a variable disease that the lung function of any individual can vary considerably from day to day, further complicating the issue of assessing clinical equivalence, particularly for preventer medicines.

Nonetheless, in spite of all these difficulties, and in spite of the previously more lenient regulatory framework, on the basis of clinical efficacy and safety, I must conclude that generic inhalers are equivalent to branded inhalers and provide a generally cheaper alternative.

David Bellamy

Dr David Bellamy, MBE, BSc, FRCP, MRCGP, is a General Practitioner in Bournemouth and a past Chairman of the GPs in Asthma Group.

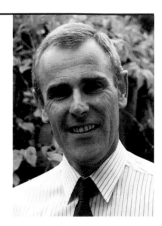

David Bellamy

74
Why should there be recognised guidelines for colour coding inhalers?

The majority of asthmatics are prescribed two different inhaler devices—a short acting β_2 agonist "reliever" inhaler and an anti-inflammatory (usually corticosteroid) "preventer" inhaler. In the well controlled patient these inhalers are taken in quite different ways. The current British Guidelines on Asthma Management suggest that a reliever should be used for symptomatic relief and prior to sport or exercise only. If the patient is symptom free they do not need to use a reliever inhaler. The preventer inhaler, on the other hand, has to be taken regularly every day, usually twice a day.

New patients and many longer standing patients may be confused as to the respective roles and frequency of use of the two types of inhaler. In consequence, the patient's use of them is ineffective and symptoms are unlikely to be properly controlled.

A lack of understanding of the action of the two types of inhaler and, particularly, that a preventer inhaler will provide no quick symptom relief are contributory factors to poor compliance with prescribed therapy. Various surveys have shown that 50–80% of patients take reliever inhalers as prescribed but that with preventers compliance levels fall to 30–50%.

In order to help both understanding and compliance with treatment, the asthma experts and pharmaceutical companies agreed a uniformity of colour coding of the two main types of inhaler devices. All types of short acting β_2 agonists, both metered dose inhalers and dry powder devices are coloured 157 blue. Beclomethasone and budesonide corticosteroid inhalers are brown, apart from Becloforte which is maroon. Of the long acting bronchodilators eformoterol has retained a light blue colour and salmeterol bright green.

The colour coding has enabled patients to differentiate more easily between groups of therapy. Colour codes can also be incorporated on written self-management plans. Using colours helps illiterate patients, the elderly, or those with poor knowledge of English to use asthma treatment more effectively.

The introduction of large numbers of generic salbutamol inhalers in the early 1990s caused much confusion as devices appeared in all sorts of colours. After much pressure from respiratory specialists a voluntary blue colour coding was introduced and most manufacturers have followed this convention. The few branded generics of beclomethasone remain brown.

The new corticosteroid fluticasone has branched into red and orange devices. Specific instructions may have to be given to patients who are changing from other brown inhalers.

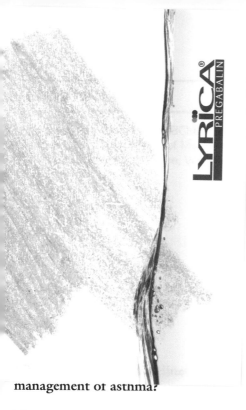

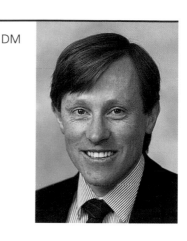

DM

...be followed for the self-management of asthma?

The majority of asthma attacks occur in the community and are self-managed by patients without immediate consultation with healthcare professionals. As a result, it is important to ensure that asthmatic patients have pre-determined written treatment guidelines to follow in the situation of an attack of asthma. For this to occur, it is necessary for patients to have the ability to recognise changes in the severity of their asthma. This can best be achieved through educating patients as to how they might perceive key symptoms that they experience and also how to interpret measurements of lung function (peak flow) that they undertake at home. With this approach, it is then possible to develop a strategy whereby treatment guidelines are recommended for patients to follow in response to changes in the severity of their asthma.

This strategy is more easily achieved through the development of an asthma self-management plan system of care that incorporates treatment guidelines. Most self-management plans have four general stages in which treatment guidelines are recommended in response to increasingly severe asthma. The stages are defined by peak flow values and a description of symptoms. The peak flow values recommended for each stage can be altered in accordance with medical preference and with the asthmatic patient's individual needs. The patient should, at all stages, administer

159

inhaled β_2 agonist therapy as required for the relief of symptoms, with an increasing frequency of use with increasingly severe asthma.

The first stage of treatment (when peak flow is 80–100% of best and symptoms are intermittent/few) provides guidelines for regular maintenance therapy, which for most patients will comprise regular inhaled corticosteroids and inhaled β_2 agonist therapy as required.

The second stage (when peak flow is 60–80% of best and there is waking at night with asthma or coughing, or symptoms suggestive of a respiratory tract infection) generally recommends an increase in the dose of inhaled corticosteroid in response to deteriorating asthma.

The third stage (when peak flow is 40–60% of best and there is increasing breathlessness or poor response to increased bronchodilator use) advises the patient to start taking oral prednisone and to contact the doctor.

The fourth stage (when peak flow is less than 40% of best) recommends seeking emergency medical treatment in this life-threatening situation.

In many respects the first two stages can be considered to provide treatment guidelines for the overall long-term management of asthma. In particular the instruction to vary the dosage of inhaled corticosteroid treatment in a stepwise manner in accordance with changes in asthma severity represents one practical method whereby the recommendations for the long-term treatment of chronic persistent asthma in adults can be implemented. As well as being advised to increase the dosage of inhaled corticosteroids in appropriate circumstances, the patient may also reduce the dose after a prolonged period of good control.

The third and fourth stages of the plan provide guidelines for the treatment of severe asthma, with intensive treatment started by the patient in an attempt to prevent the development of a life-threatening attack. Thus, treatment guidelines represent one way in which the recommendations for acute severe and chronic persistent asthma can be brought together within the framework of one system.

Since the requirements of individual asthmatic patients will vary considerably, no single self-management plan is likely to be suitable for every patient. Certain features may need to be varied. These features include the amount of detail provided; the number of stages used; the specific drug treatment recommended at each stage; and the precise level (or range of levels) of peak flow (whether pre- or post-bronchodilator) at which patients are advised to modify therapy or seek medical assistance.

One of the responsibilities now facing medical and nursing practitioners is to ensure they have the necessary knowledge and experience to produce treatment guidelines that will be practical and beneficial for the individual patients who are under their care.

Ann Woolcock

Professor Ann J. Woolcock, AO, MD, FAA, FRACP, is Professor of Respiratory Medicine at the University of Sydney, NSW, Australia.

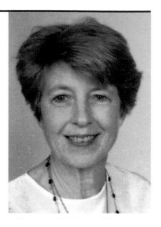

76
Should the aim of treatment be to keep asthma patients symptom free—and is this possible?

There are at least five aims of asthma treatment, the first of which is to keep the patient free from symptoms. However, for asthmatics with persistent disease, maintaining a symptom free state may not be sufficient to prevent deterioration of airway disease in the long term.

A second and important aim is therefore to achieve and maintain normal airway function. This means normal spirometric function and normal responsiveness to provoking agents such as methacholine and exercise. It is not realistic to monitor airway responsiveness on a regular basis but a good index of the degree of airway hyper-responsiveness can be obtained by measuring the peak expiratory flow rate on waking. This value should be within 10% of the best known value for peak expiratory flow and, if morning values are more than 10% below the best value, it suggests that the airway wall is thick and that the airways are hyper-responsive.

The third aim of treatment is to prevent excessive loss of lung function with time. In normal adults the forced expiratory volume in the first second of expiration (FEV_1) falls by 20 to 30 ml per year with ageing and this decrease should be the same in asthmatics. The fourth aim of treatment is to prevent death and although death is rare, it is always a risk in people with severe disease which is unrecognised or inappropriately treated. The fifth aim is to have minimal side effects of the drugs used.

By the use of an asthma self-management plan and paying attention to detail, it is possible to achieve most of these aims, in most patients, most of the time. The self-management plan is drawn up by the patient and the doctor or nurse together, and includes appropriate intervention with drugs (in particular inhaled corticosteroids), avoidance of trigger factors (where possible) and adjustment of lifestyle to include exercise, appropriate diet and avoidance of tobacco smoke. Patients with moderate or severe disease need to monitor symptoms and peak flow readings on waking and to adjust the dose of inhaled corticosteroids at regular intervals (down after a period of stable readings and up during exacerbations). In this way the dose of inhaled corticosteroids can be kept at a minimum and side effects avoided. In those with mild or episodic disease, short acting bronchodilators can be used but the use of relief medications more than three times a week indicates a requirement for the use of inhaled corticosteroids or, in children, sodium cromoglycate.

The long term use of β_2 agonists to maintain a symptom free state should be avoided because it can lead to deteriorating control of asthma.

Tim Higenbottam

Professor Tim Higenbottam, BSc, MD, MA, FRCP, is Professor of Respiratory Medicine in the Department of Medicine and Pharmacology at the University of Sheffield.

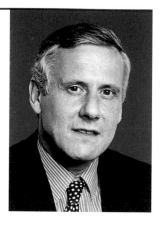

77
How can patients who continue to be breathless despite optimal treatment be managed?

The patient with asthma, when straightforward and uncomplicated, can with optimal treatment be fully restored to normal and should experience no breathlessness. Continuation of breathlessness raises four important questions, each requiring a separate area of clinical activity.

Firstly, is the treatment optimal and correct? This can be simply achieved by requesting a diary record of twice daily peak flow (PEF) measurements and bronchodilator usage, which gives an idea of asthma control. Persisting variation in PEF and high bronchodilator use suggests too little anti-inflammatory treatment. An increase of inhaled corticosteroid dose may be attempted and the diary card continued to provide an assessment of outcome. This process of evaluation of optimal treatment should also include a review of inhaler technique and a careful enquiry into compliance with medical advice.

The second question concerns aggravating factors to which the patient may be currently exposed, which are worsening the state of their asthma. Each year it has been estimated that we all experience up to five episodes of viral upper respiratory tract infections. Each, particularly the rhinovirus (common cold), can precipitate a deterioration in the asthmatic. Careful enquiry is needed, as the effects of infection can be long lasting. Action is to modify treatment temporarily, as described above when testing for the 163 optimal care. Allergen exposure at home or at work can "overwhelm" the optimal treatment of asthma. A careful enquiry is needed into occupation. For example, working in baking, in electronics or paint spraying and with animals or pets are common sources of intense allergen exposure. Referral to a specialist clinic is then advised. Also enquire into home conditions. Damp housing, old mattresses and carpets provide a home to hundreds of thousands of house dust mites. Simple avoidance approaches can be made—for example, opening bedroom windows for one hour daily to air the house and reduce humidity.

Consider alternative or additional causes of breathlessness in the patient who fails to respond. Age determines the likely alternative diagnoses. Inhaled foreign bodies in young children. The presence of emphysema or heart disease in the older asthmatic who has smoked. If these first two considerations have not provided an explanation it is appropriate to refer the patient to a specialist respiratory medicine physician.

Finally, consider inappropriate breathlessness. There are a number of asthmatics who through acute anxiety and depression or social isolation experience more symptoms than their lung function suggests. Detailed and tactful enquiry is necessary. This group with inappropriate breathlessness again require diary card review of PEF together with counselling and advice. Remember that this group has the potential to abuse therapy, corticosteroids and bronchodilators. Through such action they can cause themselves harm. They also can be frequent clinic attenders. For those with psychiatric illness referral to a psychiatric specialist is important.

Remember asthma is an illness that can vary enormously in intensity. Good advice on PEF monitoring should pick up early the developing acute asthma attack.

Anthony Newman Taylor

Professor Anthony Newman Taylor, OBE, MSC, FRCP, FFOM, is Professor of Occupational and Environmental Medicine at the National Heart and Lung Institute, Imperial College of Science, Technology and Medicine, London and Consultant Physician at the Royal Brompton Hospital, London. He is Chairman of the Industrial Injuries Advisory Council at the Department of Social Security.

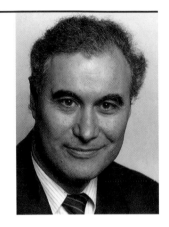

78
How can occupational asthma be managed?

Asthma due to the development of allergy to a substance inhaled at work is important to identify because, being caused by a single specific agent encountered in a particular environment (the workplace), it represents one of the few occasions when asthma in adults can be improved or cured. Equally, however, because such improvement requires avoidance of further exposure to the cause, which can require a change of job, incorrect attribution of asthma to occupational allergy can have disastrous financial and social consequences. Mis-diagnosis can be as harmful as missing the diagnosis.

Management of occupational asthma is based on good evidence that asthma was initiated by a substance at work, accurate identification of the specific cause and avoidance of further exposure to it. Avoidance of exposure can be achieved in the following ways:

- Substitution of the specific cause of asthma by another less hazardous material (unusual—but occasionally achieved).
- Segregation and enclosure of the hazardous process, allowing the affected individual to avoid exposure to the cause.
- Relocation of the individual to another part of the workplace where not exposed to the cause of asthma.
- Wearing of respiratory protection equipment (RPE)—such as laminar flow equipment— when in contact with the cause of asthma. RPE is of   165

particular value for dusts that cause occupational asthma—such as laboratory animal secreta and excreta and drugs such as antibiotics.

- Leaving the workplace. Unfortunately this can sometimes be the only means by which those affected are able to avoid exposure to the cause of their asthma. This is particularly true in small factories where opportunities for adequate relocation can be very limited.

Studies of occupational asthma caused by several agents, including isocyanates, colophony, Western Red Cedar dust and acid anhydrides, have shown that asthma and airway hyper-responsiveness, although improved after avoidance of exposure to their cause, in about 50% of cases do not resolve. This seems particularly to occur to individuals who have remained exposed to the cause of their asthma for prolonged periods after its onset. Surveillance in workplaces where causes of asthma are present should, therefore, focus on the early identification of asthma, and on confirmation of its cause, in order to allow early avoidance of exposure and the maximum probability of resolution of asthma.

Peter Calverley

Professor Peter M.A. Calverley, MB ChB, FRCP, FCCP, is Professor of Medicine (Pulmonary Rehabilitation) at the University of Liverpool and Consultant Physician at Fazakerley Hospital, Liverpool.

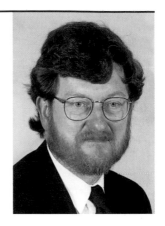

79
What is the influence of smoking on asthma?

Cigarette smoking is a major cause of avoidable ill health throughout the world. There is compelling evidence that smoking is the principal cause in older people of chronic obstructive lung disease (COLD), also known as chronic obstructive pulmonary disease (COPD), which is frequently confused with asthma. However, there is no evidence that smoking is a major direct cause of asthma in younger people nor that it increases the death rate among asthmatics. In fact, many older asthmatics may remember using or being told of herbal "asthma cigarettes" which contain the plant equivalent of the modern drug ipratropium bromide (Atrovent) and which were sold over the counter to asthma sufferers.

However, new knowledge has led to a reconsideration of the traditionally neutral attitude towards asthmatics who smoke. Studies of young families have shown that children whose parents smoke are almost twice as likely to develop asthma as those brought up in a non-smoking household. There is even more powerful evidence that mothers who smoke during the first six months of their pregnancy are much more likely to give birth to a child who will develop asthma. Sadly, many more young women now smoke and find it harder to give up than their male contemporaries. Maternal smoking may be an important factor in the increasing incidence of asthma in children.

Why this should happen is not clear but changes to the child's immune responses in utero seem a likely explanation. Smoking in adults is known to 167 be associated with a raised eosinophil count and a greater risk of atopy which may improve when the person stops using cigarettes. There is growing evidence that some smokers who develop COLD are more likely to have irritable airways when younger and to have inflammatory changes in their airways which are related to those seen in young asthmatics. Interestingly, these changes do not completely resolve when the smoker stops but may improve when inhaled corticosteroids are given. Some smokers develop an asthma-like illness when they give up but the symptoms of this increased reactivity will usually slowly disappear. Their rate of disappearance can be improved by a short period of inhaled corticosteroid treatment, but unlike true asthmatics, these symptoms do not recur when the corticosteroid is stopped. There is still a lot to learn about the connections between asthma and chronic lung disease and the role which smoking plays in producing them.

Cigarette smoke contains many chemicals and particles which irritate the airways. Smokers are more likely to cough and develop respiratory tract infections than are non-smokers, both being troublesome problems for someone with asthma. Many asthma specialists suspect that smokers respond less well to anti-asthma treatment and have poorer asthma control than do non-smokers, although this is yet to be scientifically established. Moreover, smoking asthmatics may be more likely to go on to fixed airways obstruction. For all these reasons, and more, smoking is not good for asthmatics and should be strongly discouraged. Help with giving up smoking, including the use of nicotine patches and joining support groups, can be a good long-term investment in the asthma patient's future health.

Ronald Dahl

Professor Ronald Dahl, MD, is Professor of
Respiratory Diseases and Allergy, Arhus
University Hospital, Denmark.

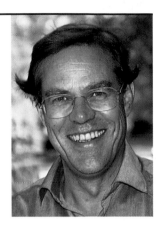

80
What steps can be taken to help asthma patients to give up smoking?

It is important that all healthcare professionals have a clear opinion about the dangers of smoking and are able to express their concern convincingly.

Asthmatics need to be told that they are especially vulnerable to the acute effects of tobacco smoke. Inhaled tobacco is a major trigger factor in asthma, inducing acute bronchospasm and mucus production. This can be demonstrated to patients. Some need to be told that the expectoration caused by smoking is not helpful. They may be clearing their airways but they are clearing only newly produced, tobacco induced secretions.

Asthmatics also need to know that smoking will hasten the development of long-term problems, such as chronic obstructive pulmonary disease (COPD). It is very difficult, and may be impossible, to relieve asthma symptoms and asthma disease progression in an asthmatic who smokes. Asthma medications are less effective and may seem useless. This makes therapeutic decisions even more difficult because it raises the question of whether it is acceptable to prescribe expensive and potentially dangerous medications to make it tolerable for an asthmatic to smoke.

Most asthmatic smokers would like to quit but need support and advice. They need to know that it often takes more than one attempt to give up smoking permanently and that success will depend on their own will to quit. Different helping strategies are needed depending on a patient's age, knowledge, health beliefs, etc. For teenagers, it can be helpful to organise a 169 group discussion with other asthmatics of the same age, not necessarily smokers. Arguments for giving up smoking that often appeal to this age group are those relating to physical fitness and personal appearance. Among the next age group, young adults, an important argument is the adverse effect of passive smoking on children, especially on children with an inherited predisposition to develop asthma. In older age groups, the effect of smoking on life expectancy and daily activities are accepted arguments. At all ages, giving up smoking has advantages relating to health, personal finances, safety and the environment.

For asthmatics, as for all smokers wanting to quit, it is very important to prepare properly and to set a date for giving up. In the preparation phase it is necessary that the asthmatic is convinced that this is the most important project that he or she is engaged in this year, and that he or she is certain, confident and mentally determined to quit. The asthmatic should seek support from family, friends and colleagues and ask for their praise. If the asthmatic's partner smokes it is an advantage if both can decide to give up smoking together. It may also be useful to make a contract and to read information materials about stopping smoking.

Before quitting, the asthmatic smoker should evaluate his or her degree of addiction and discuss whether there is a need for a period of nicotine substitution. He or she should also consider measures against possible weight gain, including changes to diet and exercise patterns. It can also be useful to start a new project, such as a hobby, educational programme, home renovation or work in the garden. Another idea is to make it more and more difficult to smoke in this preparation period, by imposing self-inflicted limits on when and where smoking is allowed.

In the period before and after giving up smoking, the asthmatic should keep a diary with peak flow measurements morning and evening and an evaluation of day- and night-time symptoms. Possible problems can also be written down for future discussion. The doctor and nurse should be fully engaged in the preparation phase and also after the patient stops smoking. Frequent and regular follow-up is needed to support continued abstinence from smoking. It can also be useful for the patient to join a group of other people who are giving up smoking.

Healthcare professionals should always express a strong and continued interest in smoking cessation and should encourage and help patients to prepare to quit. This is in no way different from the problem of smoking cessation in any smoker, but the asthmatic should know that he or she is at special risk and that asthma may be impossible to control by the usual means in persistent smokers. An individual approach should always be tried depending on the individual's own needs.

Malcolm Green

Dr Malcolm Green, DM, FRCP, is Consultant
Physician at the Royal Brompton Hospital,
London.

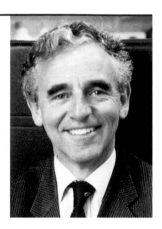

81
What is the planned phase-out of inhalers containing CFCs?

Metered dose inhalers (MDIs) were introduced in the 1950s and have been
a mainstay of the treatment of asthma since that time. Indeed there are now
450 million MDIs prescribed worldwide every year. The patients who use
them find them convenient, and they are tried and tested. Although the
inhalers are technically sophisticated, the technology itself is not expensive.
However, there is a problem: MDIs use chloro-fluoro-carbons (CFCs) as
the propellant. Following the implication of CFCs in the destruction of the
ozone layer, production of these chemicals is currently being phased out
by international agreement, under the terms of the so-called Montreal
Protocol and its updates. Production of CFCs ceased in the European
Union in January 1995 and across the rest of the world in January 1996, for
all purposes with one significant exception, that of MDIs. So effective has
this phase-out been that MDIs are now responsible for 95% of the production of CFCs in Europe. Thus, on the one hand, MDIs are invaluable for
the management of asthma, but on the other, they are destroying the health
of the ozone layer.

For this reason the pharmaceutical industry has been actively developing
CFC-free inhalers over the last five years or so. Technically this is a difficult
challenge as it requires substantial redesign of many of the parts of the
inhalers, including their valves and sealants as well as the propellant itself.
Most, if not all, companies have decided to use a new substance, HFA134A,   171

as the CFC-free propellant, and intensive research has shown this to be extremely safe. It is degraded in the atmosphere long before it reaches the ozone layer and it contains no damaging chlorine molecules. One company has already introduced to the market a CFC-free salbutamol inhaler which is available on prescription. It seems likely that other medications and CFC-free inhalers will become available over the next year or two. Hopefully by the end of 1997 patients in the UK will be able to convert from their current inhalers to similar CFC-free inhalers.

The Montreal Protocol requires any exemptions to be justified annually, and in June 1996 the exemption panel decided that the process should be speeded up for MDIs. It was therefore recommended that no further new CFC-containing inhalers should be licensed, and that the vast majority of CFC-containing inhalers be phased out by the year 2000, with an absolute ban by the year 2005. The panel will, however, review these dates annually, and anticipates being able to shorten the timescale provided the new inhalers come on stream as predicted.

This change is of great importance for health professionals and patients alike. It means that, in effect, all patients will have to change their inhalers within the next three years. The transition will not be easy as both health professionals and patients will have to become used to the new inhalers, which may be slightly different in shape, sensation and strength. Evidence from the US suggests, however, that patients rapidly become happy with their new inhalers, and find little difficulty in the changeover, at least with the salbutamol inhaler so far available. However, health professionals and purchasers will need to devise a strategy for the changeover, and will have to decide whether patients should be changed one inhaler at a time as they become available, or should wait until two or three inhalers are on the market. They will have to work out how to discuss this with each patient and effect and monitor the change. This process will be time-consuming and will need to be carefully planned. Purchasers and pharmacists will need to be involved in deciding which of the new products should be provided in a given hospital or area, and this will need to match with the requirements of prescribers and patients alike.

It is vital that the respiratory community and patients should co-operate actively in this important new change. Our children will not thank us if we continue to damage the ozone layer a minute longer than is necessary. Even now, the damage will not be repaired until the end of the next century and so the continued use of CFCs is not sustainable, and will not be allowed by international convention. Over the next year or two CFC-containing MDIs will no longer be available and the transition will need to be complete by the end of 1999. This is a challenge for us all.

Donald Lane

Dr Donald Lane, DM, FRCP, is Consultant
Physician at the Osler Chest Unit, Churchill
Hospital, Oxford.

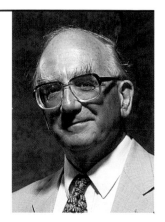

82
What is the place of complementary therapy in the treatment of asthma?

Since the treatment of asthma with conventional inhaled therapy is so obviously successful, it might well be questioned whether any form of complementary treatment is ever worth consideration. But there are three scenarios where its use is often raised: when conventional therapy fails to control the asthma; when conventional therapy causes unpleasant or dangerous side effects; when the patient requests its use.

Before proposing complementary therapy in the above settings, we should satisfy ourselves that prescribed conventional therapy is being taken properly, regularly and in an appropriate dose; that reported unwanted effects are genuine and likely to be due to the medication; and that all misunderstandings about the prescribed therapy have been cleared up. It must also be insisted that the treatment chosen is seen truly as "complementary" and not as "alternative". The sudden abandonment of standard treatment is potentially dangerous.

So what is on offer? Closest to conventional medicine is herbal medicine. This cannot be recommended, offering nothing more than unidentified, unstandardised, unpurified versions of what might be conventional therapy if properly processed. Sodium cromoglycate started life in this way. Some herbal remedies contain corticosteroid-like substances and some dangerous toxins. There is an overwhelming case for 173 the regulation of herbal remedies, licensing them for use in the same way as conventional drug therapy.

Homeopathy employs solutions of therapies so dilute that they are devoid of activity in a conventional pharmacologic sense. Properly controlled trials in asthma are few and not convincing.

Stemming from traditional breathing exercises is a whole range of physical therapies that may help under specific circumstances. In the sense that asthma induces panic, and panic leads to hyperventilation, which can itself make asthma worse, any technique that fosters appropriate control over the rate and depth of breathing can be valuable. This is, however, control over skeletal muscle in the thorax not over the smooth muscle of the bronchial tree. Yet one study of a specialised yoga technique, called pranayama breathing, did appear to show that it reduced bronchial hyper-reactivity. The practitioners of osteopathy and chiropractic also claim that spinal manipulation can relax bronchial smooth muscle. This is more likely to work, when it does, through relaxing thoracic cage tension, particularly that caused by hyper-inflation. Individual patients report benefit. There have been no satisfactory trials.

There are several studies showing that appropriate suggestion can cause both bronchodilatation and bronchoconstriction. Harnessing this for benefit is difficult. It is most evident in hypnosis. Some remarkable claims have been made for hypnosis. It has never been widely used in asthma but some studies by dedicated hypnotists seem convincing. To make the technique practical, patients are taught self-hypnosis. Doubts have, however, been expressed about the safety of this—the fear being that it might obscure the ability to recognise an impending severe attack.

Acupuncture, though part of a therapeutic culture alien to the Western world, may also ultimately be shown to act through the nervous system, either by the direct stimulation of autonomic nerves or through the release of central endogenous peptides. Some of the best studies of any complementary therapy are those using acupuncture for asthma. Appropriate and quite specific needling have been shown to produce short-term bronchodilatation, but convincing evidence of long-term sustained benefit is difficult to come by.

If you contemplate recommending a complementary therapy, ensure your own confidence in the practitioner and preferably stick to those regulated by a professional body—or, if you choose to carry out a therapy yourself, get properly trained. Do not dabble and do make objective observations of the effects you achieve.

Chapter 5

Asthma Education: For patients and professionals

Liesl Osman

Dr L.M. Osman, PhD, Reg Psych, is NAC Senior
Research Fellow in the Organisation of Asthma
Care at the Department of Medicine and
Therapeutics, University of Aberdeen and at the
Chest Clinic, City Hospital, Aberdeen.

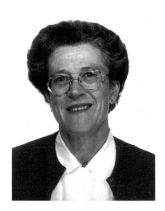

83
What basic asthma education should be given to all asthma patients?

A diagnosis of asthma can be a relief. The patient (or patient's parent) can
feel that the doctor now knows what will help them. But every patient will
bring their own reactions and expectations to the idea that they have
asthma. Equally, much of what the doctor or nurse knows and takes for
granted may be quite difficult for the patient to grasp and remember.

When we talk to patients with asthma we find many people who do not
know the difference between their preventive and relief inhalers even after
months or years of use, who do not feel in control of their asthma, and who
use ineffective strategies to manage their asthma. For these people something has not gone well in the process of learning what asthma is and how to
manage it. Asthma education aims to enable the patient:

- to know what to do for their own asthma management and how to do it
  (medication instructions, inhaler technique);
- to agree that following these instructions and advice is worthwhile
  (questions and anxieties have been raised and answered);
- to feel comfortable with saying to you, their doctor or nurse, that their
  management is not working well for them (good interaction and discussion of what the patient does to help themselves);
- to understand why they need to visit a doctor or nurse when feeling well
  (chronic illness controlled through review and care when well, not
  through crisis management). 177

After an asthma diagnosis all sorts of fundamental questions may be important to the patient but never answered by the health professional. The whole process of review is likely to be a new idea to the patient. Most of us visit a doctor only when we are ill. Most of us normally use medicine to control symptoms, not to prevent them. Basic asthma education recognises that patients may be quite bewildered by the whole new situation that this diagnosis has introduced. Also, it needs to be recognised that medical information is difficult for most people to take in and remember at the best of times.

The key steps in basic asthma education for patients are as follows:

- Explain why you have decided on the diagnosis of asthma (e.g., because an inhaled corticosteroid trial has helped their symptoms). Give the patient time to ask questions about what asthma means.
- Discuss the patient's current symptoms, what they find helps, and how their new medication will help. Emphasise that their preventive medicine will reduce the need to use relief medication.
- Clearly state (in a written self-management plan) how often the patient should take their inhaled corticosteroid (use the name the patient will see on the prescription). Clearly state what you have both decided is normal use for them of their relief inhaler. Explain that increased use of their relief inhaler is a sign that more preventive control is needed.
- Acknowledge that people sometimes have concerns about using medication regularly, or using inhaled corticosteroids. Let them express these concerns, if they have them, and reassure them with concrete evidence that their medication is not harmful.
- Discuss possible lifestyle changes. You may want to emphasise that the most helpful lifestyle change is to stop smoking.
- Check that they are happy with their inhaler and that they are confident how to use it.
- Emphasise that it is absolutely possible to lead a full and vigorous life with well controlled asthma.

The three principles of successful basic asthma education for patients can be summarised as "three Ps and one R". To expand on this: each patient's asthma education programme needs to be Personalised, Practical, Preventive and Repeated.

Mac Cochrane

Dr G.M. Cochrane, BSc, MB, BS, FRCP, is
Consultant Physician, Honorary Senior Lecturer
and Postgraduate Dean at Guy's Hospital,
London.

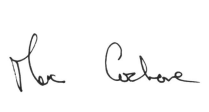

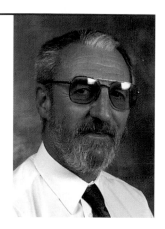

84
What is the degree of compliance in asthma management?

Compliance or adherence is defined as the extent to which a person's behaviour (in terms of taking medication or making dietary or lifestyle changes) coincides with advice from healthcare professionals. Such a definition assumes that the correct diagnosis has been made, that the healthcare professional's advice is appropriate and that the patient is able to follow the advice. Over 20 years ago, surveys of asthma deaths suggested that these deaths were associated with failure to diagnose the severity of the disease and with failure to give sound advice. More recently, similar surveys have suggested that both asthma mortality and morbidity are now associated with a failure of patients to comply, rather than with their having been given poor advice.

There are, of course, different types of non-compliance. Let us look first at attendances at clinics and hospital Accident and Emergency (A&E) Departments. Of attendances at A&E for acute severe asthma, up to 15% are made by patients who have run out of their prophylactic medication in the previous month. Almost a third are by patients who have failed to seek advice from their general practitioners despite the acute attack having lasted for two to three days. Follow-up appointments arranged at the time of the A&E visit to take place at a hospital chest clinic or the patient's general practice are not kept by over a quarter of these patients. Failure to attend regularly at asthma clinics, either in the 179 community or at the hospital, is the ultimate form of non-compliance and can be as high as 25% in inner cities.

There are also clearly problems with compliance relating to recommended changes to lifestyle. Asthmatics are frequently advised to change their local environment, such as by changing feather pillows and duvets, or by getting rid of pets such as cats. Although there are few formal studies, advice of this type is frequently not followed, generally because it is, in the view of the patient, inappropriate or impossible. In one meta analysis, however, the authors demonstrated that although only 28% of patients complied with environmental advice when instructed by their general practitioners, the level of compliance could rise to 62% if a group education approach was used. Lifestyle changes such as stopping smoking or losing weight are clearly seldom followed, as can be seen from the fact that up to 30% of asthmatics continue to smoke!

Let us look finally at patient compliance with therapy. The extent of compliance with oral and inhaled therapy has been difficult to assess, particularly as until recently there were few accurate assessment techniques. The doctors' impression has been shown to be inaccurate, and asking the patient about his or her level of compliance is inevitably associated with considerable over-estimation. Although spot blood tests can be used to identify non-compliance with theophyllines, these tests also over-estimate compliance levels. The recent introduction of electronic devices recording the time of actuation or inspiration of drugs has suggested the following compliance levels in patients on twice daily prophylaxis. About a third of patients regularly take almost all their inhaled therapy, a further third probably take over 50% of their prescribed medication, whereas the remaining third take little or no medication. Compliance with oral medication (if on a twice daily regimen) in asthmatics is said to be greater than with inhaled prophylactic therapy, but there are as yet no studies comparing oral anti-asthma prophylaxis using the new leukotriene antagonists.

David Pendleton

Dr David Pendleton, D Phil, AFBPsS, C Psychol, is a Director of Opus Consulting, Bristol.

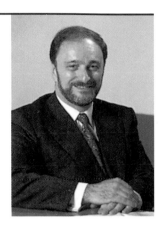

85
What factors affect compliance?

It is frustrating to think that so much sound medical advice is wasted. The best estimate is that about a third of medical advice is followed accurately, a third is rejected, and a third is followed inaccurately. So there are two forms of non-compliance—witting and unwitting. Each has been studied extensively and we understand both quite well. The factors affecting each form of non-compliance are, naturally, different.

In the case of unwitting non-compliance, the patient is simply getting it wrong in some way. In the case of asthma medication, the patient has to remember the difference between preventers and relievers, on demand versus regular medication schedules, and the colours of the inhalers. In the case of more complex medication, the situation worsens.

The principle causes of unwitting non-compliance come down to two factors: memory and understanding. My own research indicated that patients' memory for medication advice was really quite good but that, naturally, simpler advice is easier to remember than more complex advice, and simpler treatment regimes are likely to be followed better.

Understanding can be a major problem, by contrast. Most doctors and nurses over-estimate how much medical information their patients understand, and many information leaflets are written at too high a level for widespread understanding. They should be picked carefully with the reading age of the patient in mind.

181

The more difficult problems concern the rejection of advice—the aspects of witting non-compliance. Two factors stand out: patients' ideas, and the communication between doctor and patient.

As regards the first of these factors, patients' ideas, patients are actively thinking about their condition when they come to the surgery. They may have learned not to say much to a busy-looking doctor or nurse, but they have a vested interest in their health and think about it often. If the doctor or nurse offers advice that is inconsistent with the patient's beliefs, they have a struggle to fit it all together and may reject the advice given, preferring their own ideas. If, for example, they believe that they can build up their own resistance to the house dust mite by increasing their exposure to it, then preventer medication may be rejected.

The key here is to ensure that time is made to discuss the patient's ideas in the consultation. These ideas can then be either reinforced or discussed. Of particular impact are the patient's beliefs about the seriousness of his or her condition and how it might need to be treated. Expectations of how the doctor or nurse might handle the matter are also useful to consider together with the patient.

Additionally, some patients have become fatalistic about their health and genuinely do not believe that they can do much about it. These patients need to be shown ways in which their health can be positively affected by their own efforts.

The second major factor in witting non-compliance is doctor–patient communication. When decisions are made *for* patients, they are often rejected. When decisions are made *with* patients, they are more often followed. Authoritarian consulting tends not to work. In order for patients to follow advice well, they need to be fully involved at all stages of the consultation: diagnosis, management and treatment.

Similarly, when patients believe that the advice they have been given has been tailored just to their own needs and lifestyle, rather than being generally given to most patients similarly, they tend to follow the advice.

So, in summary, the factors that affect compliance are as follows:

- Patients' memory and understanding.
- Patients' ideas and beliefs.
- The extent to which the patient is involved in the consultation.
- General or tailored advice given by the doctor or nurse.

Kenneth Chapman

Dr Kenneth R. Chapman, MD, MSc, FRCPC, FACP, is Director of the Asthma Centre of the Toronto Hospital and Associate Professor of Medicine at the University of Toronto, Ontario, Canada.

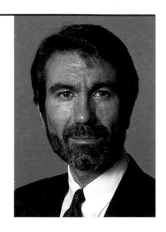

86
How does asthma education improve compliance?

We would all like to believe that education of the patient improves compliance with prescribed therapy. The classic scenario is of a patient whose asthma is poorly controlled for lack of compliance with a prescribed inhaled corticosteroid. Perhaps the patient fears the use of steroids or perhaps fails to distinguish between bronchodilator and preventive therapy. Perhaps sub-optimal compliance is inadvertent and results from poor inhaler technique. Education is offered, the patient's confusion is dispelled and the consequent improvement in compliance results in better asthma control. Unfortunately, we have little direct research evidence to show that education works reliably to produce this effect and there is ample reason to believe that the scenario is an over-simplification.

For most healthcare professionals, compliance is seen as a problem of medication under-use. Although this is the most common form of poor compliance, compliance problems may also take the form of medication over-use or erratic compliance (when the patient complies with therapy only intermittently). Intelligent non-compliance is a term used to describe patients who make a reasoned choice not to use the prescribed therapy as recommended—often for good reason (e.g. the patient with mild asthma who declines a prescription for β_2 agonist inhalation). There are many factors that lead to these patterns of less than perfect compliance; socio-economic factors are key among them. No amount of education can result 183 in compliance with a high-dose and high-cost inhaled corticosteroid therapy if the patient is unable to pay for the prescription. Cultural beliefs may cause the patient to reject information delivered by a physician or healthcare professional of a different ethnic or cultural background. Impaired family cohesiveness has been recognised as a common cause of sub-optimal compliance with therapy in asthmatic children; if no single family member is reliably responsible for giving medication to a child, compliance with therapy will be sub-optimal. Adolescent "rebellion" may lead to deliberate non-compliance with medication as the teenager attempts to establish his or her own autonomy.

Surprisingly little research in patient education has used objective monitoring of drug use to assess compliance. Almost all research uses patient self-reporting, a notoriously unreliable means of assessing true compliance. Although some published research suggests that patient education improves compliance, it may be simply that the educated patient knows the "correct" answer and provides it when prompted. In a striking example of patients giving the answer that is expected of them, researchers of the US National Institute of Health "Lung Health Study" compared patient diary records of thrice daily inhaler use to Chronolog records of actual inhaler use. (The Chronolog is an electronic device that records not only the number of actuations of aerosol canister but the date and time the actuations were made.) Not surprisingly, diary records regularly over-estimated actual use. When researchers reviewed the electronic recording from the Chronologs, they were astonished to discover a large number of patients repeatedly actuating their canisters scores of times just before their clinic visits so as to present the façade of optimal compliance.

In summary, effective education can break down some but not all of the barriers to optimal patient compliance. Future research should employ objective monitoring techniques to examine the impact of education on patient compliance.

Mike Ward

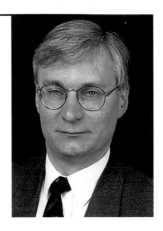

Dr Mike Ward, MB ChB (Hons), MRCP, is Consultant Physician and Executive Medical Director at King's Mill Centre for Health Care Services, Mansfield, Nottinghamshire.

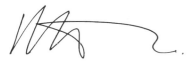

87
Does asthma education reduce morbidity and mortality?

Surveys of asthma morbidity carried out in 1989 in the United Kingdom demonstrated that many asthmatics required time off work or school because of their asthma and were frequently awake at night with cough and wheeze. A survey in 1996 indicated that for the asthmatic population as a whole things have not changed, despite the ever-increasing prescription of bronchodilators and inhaled anti-inflammatories. The 1996 survey reported that:

- 43% of asthmatics were woken at night at least once a week by cough or wheeze;
- 25% had at least one week off school because of asthma in the previous year;
- 41% experienced symptoms most days;
- 25% felt asthma totally controlled their life or had a major effect on it.

Reports have highlighted problems such as lack of patient knowledge about asthma treatments, delays in seeking help and incorrect self-management decisions. This led to consideration of the question of whether asthma education can change patient behaviour and improve morbidity and mortality?

The first papers researching the place of patient education in asthma used patient interviews, education leaflets and audiotapes. These "gave" the patient information but failed to improve asthma morbidity, with no effect on night-time wakening, on time off school or work or on the frequency of asthma attacks. There are now similar studies in asthma, diabetes and hypertension showing that improving patient knowledge on its own does not improve morbidity or mortality. In the 1990s, therefore, asthma education changed emphasis, moving away from "improving knowledge" towards involving the patient in an agreed self-management plan. Such plans use written information to give the patient instruction about what to do when asthma is well-controlled or deteriorating. The plans mostly involve three steps: increased inhaled corticosteroids, use of oral cortico-steroids and urgent medical attention.

In adults, self-management plans have produced a reduction in asthma morbidity, with less night take wakening, less time off work and fewer acute exacerbations. The use of self-management plans in children, however, has not been as promising. A recent analysis of 11 self-management teaching programmes suggested that the self-management plan did not seem to reduce morbidity.

The following questions still remain to be addressed. If self-management plans are effective, why is asthma morbidity the same in 1996 as it was in 1989, and why might they not be as effective in children. I think the answer to these questions is that self-management plans should be viewed as only part of an "asthma education programme". We know that only 50% of patients comply with medication, and it is naïve to think that written instructions given to patients will on their own mean that the patient will ignore their own beliefs or goals. Education programmes must use self-management plans along with good communication skills to involve the patient in a partnership to identify and satisfy the specific needs of the patient as perceived by that patient, not only those thought to be important by the doctor or nurse.

Studies in parts of the United Kingdom have shown that asthma education using self-management plans has improved morbidity. It is likely that morbidity for asthma in the country as a whole will improve if more nurses and doctors are trained to use them. Self-management plans should be part of a broader asthma education programme which also utilises other skills to produce a satisfied patient.

Julian Crane

Dr Julian Crane, FRACP, MRCP (UK),
Dip Comm H, is Health Research Council
Professorial Research Fellow and Medical
Director of the Asthma & Respiratory
Foundation of New Zealand.

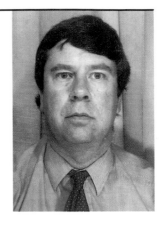

88
What is the role of self-management plans in asthma care?

The modern concept of asthma self-management stems from the notion of greater autonomy, self responsibility and self reliance for patients with asthma, while continuing to recognise the importance of advice and information from health professionals—the concept of partnership: "The patient takes the helm, health professionals chart the course". In addition to this idea, asthma self-management plans have been developed to:
- improve an individual's asthma management;
- increase knowledge and awareness about asthma and its treatment;
- improve asthma morbidity and mortality.

All individuals with asthma who have treatment prescribed for them have always undertaken self-management based on their perceived symptom severity. The concept of systematically organising self-management into a series of straightforward written assessment and treatment instructions is new. Most plans incorporate two important elements: the objective assessment of lung function by self-measurement of peak flow, and the taking of therapeutic actions based on this assessment.

This new notion of self-management grew directly from concerns in the 1980s that mortality and morbidity were rising. Studies of asthma mortality suggested that patients often died because they delayed seeking help, under-estimating their own asthma severity, and because they, their family or friends and often health professionals failed to appreciate the severity of   187 their final attack. To underline this, laboratory studies have suggested that some patients with asthma are simply unaware of just how poor their lung function is, reporting their breathing as "good" or "normal" when they have peak flow recordings less than half of their predicted value.

A number of questions about self-management plans still remain. First we need to ask why studies examining the effect of self-management plans on morbidity have given conflicting results. I suspect that the conflicting results on reducing morbidity arise largely because of differences in management before the plans are introduced. If patients are already being well managed there is little room for improvement. If they are not, then the introduction of self-management and the education necessary to undertake it effectively, will improve their asthma. Indeed, studies have clearly demonstrated such an improvement.

The next question is whether all patients with asthma should have a self-management plan. The answer to this is that patients with recurrent or continual symptoms requiring regular high dose anti-inflammatory treatment should have a plan, a peak flow meter and a supply of oral corticosteroids to use in the event of a severe deterioration. On the other hand the patient with occasional wheezing who uses bronchodilators alone, probably does not require a detailed plan or a peak flow meter. For patients between these extremes it is a matter of clinical judgement for the patient and their adviser. Even when there is little objective improvement in morbidity, the increased confidence and self reliance that self-management gives to patients seems well worth the effort.

Finally we should consider what might be the optimum treatment advice and settings of PEF for management plans. These will vary from country to country and from patient to patient, and will change with growing experience and improvements in asthma therapy. It is important that the use and efficacy of management plans is regularly examined and updated. In the end the patient will decide if he or she wishes to continue steering the ship, at present most patients should be given the option.

Ian Charlton

Dr Ian Charlton, MBBS, MRCGP, is a General Practitioner in Kincumber, NSW, Australia and the Founding Chairman of the Australian GPs in Asthma Group.

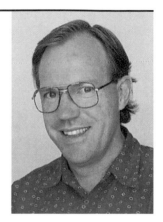

89
Should every patient who is managed in general practice have a home peak flow meter?

The brief answer to this question is "No", but that up to half of patients with asthma would benefit from home peak flow monitoring providing that appropriate training were available.

Peak flow meters alone will not improve self-management in asthma care. The key issue is the need for patients to understand the significance of their symptoms and what actions they should take. Learning this process can be greatly enhanced by the use of a peak flow meter, although training of patients does take several months.

A peak flow meter will be of little value to patients who experience occasional mild symptoms. These patients are unlikely to remember how to interpret their results. Many of the peak flow meters issued to these patients have a habit of being "lost".

Current reports suggest that up to 60% of patients in general practice are prescribed prophylactic therapy. These patients would be experiencing frequent and troublesome symptoms and should be assessed as to whether they may benefit from using a peak flow meter. It is at this point that patients may recognise the benefits in terms of reduced morbidity against the cost and inconvenience of monitoring.

Many patients may be able to manage their asthma based on symptoms alone, particularly if a collection of symptoms is used and then compiled   189 into a symptom score. This works well for patients who are too old or too young to use a meter. However, a large group of patients are "poor perceivers" and are therefore not able to identify physical symptoms as warnings of deteriorating lung function. There is no ready way of identifying poor perceivers. Unfortunately, doctors have also been found wanting in making an accurate assessment of the severity of a patient's asthma. The peak flow meter offers both sides of the consultation the opportunity of quantifying asthma in a manner that can be easily interpreted.

The peak flow reading is a measure of tracheal diameter and is not as accurate as spirometry in measuring small to medium size airway calibre. Studies have highlighted that peak flow recordings on their own can be unreliable in assessing the severity of asthma. Similarly, the use of single symptoms has been found inadequate. However, peak flow meters can greatly enhance the teaching of self-management skills when they are used as a training tool in conjunction with patient monitoring of a collection of symptoms and medication usage. This training can be reinforced by the use of colour coded stickers on the meter which give appropriate instructions to be followed when the readings fall.

The peak flow meter needs to be "sold" to the patient. There is often a "window of opportunity" when patients may be ready to accept the need for a peak flow meter and the training that goes with it. Patients who have attended asthma education programmes can take three months before they are confident to use a peak flow meter, interpret the results and implement appropriate self-management strategies. Amongst this group of patients, 25% use the peak flow meter every day, 20% use them weekly, 45% use them only with an attack and 10% do not use them at all.

Several studies have suggested peak flow meters should be issued to patients with severe disease. These studies were performed in hospital-based patients. Self-management plans enabling the patient to take action before the attack developed, for example by doubling the dose of inhaled corticosteroid, were not used.

It is worth noting as a final point that asthma morbidity can be halved when peak flow meters are used in conjunction with training programmes and appropriately structured self-management plans and strategies that help patients to understand the significance of their symptoms.

Frankie Brown

Frankie Brown, SRN, OND, NATC Dip in Asthma Care, is Lecturer Practitioner (General Practice) at Brookes University, Oxford and a National Asthma Training Centre Regional Trainer.

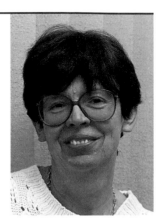

90
What skills are required to improve asthma consultations?

Healthcare professionals involved in asthma consultations, both organised and opportunistic, need to look carefully at communication skills. Without good communication skills, up-to-date medical knowledge is meaningless because patients do not benefit from it. Every effort is needed to give patients clear explanations and to avoid medical jargon.

It is also necessary to have a genuine interest in the patient and his or her asthma in order to become aware of each patient's own perceived and actual needs. This involves the healthcare professional in seeking a greater understanding of the patient's attitude towards, and concerns about, his or her condition as well as in developing skills that will encourage patients to tell us about their personal health beliefs. Such beliefs can have a profound effect on a patient's attitude to diagnosis and to interventions by doctors or nurses. Advice which is geared explicitly to a patient's current ideas and needs will generally be more readily acceptable. As Sir William Osler said: "It is more important to know what sort of patient has a disease than what sort of disease a patient has".

The skill of time management is also valuable during asthma consultations. A consultation can be more effective if healthcare professional and patient agree in advance about what they want to talk about and what priority they should give to the various topics. Once this has been achieved, it is possible to move forward at the patient's pace, exploring   191 techniques for helping him or her to make constructive changes for improving asthma control.

Listening is a key skill in good communication, but it needs to be active not passive. Body position and eye contact, as well as the setting in which the consultation takes place, all have a part to play in encouraging the patient to communicate. Active listening also involves carefully watching the patient, who will often communicate clues non-verbally, such as by reacting apprehensively to a particular piece of information.

During consultations it is important to ask "open" questions, which generally invite longer replies than closed questions, which can be answered in a word or two, such as by a simple "yes" or "no". Open questions are very useful for encouraging patients to ask questions of their own. Closed questions can, however, also have a place in the consultation, where it is necessary to ask patients for quite specific information.

The patient needs always to be shown support and understanding for the way he or she feels. Comments along the lines of "I can see why you might be unsure of that" can be helpful. An indirect approach, such as "Do you know anyone else who has asthma, have you talked to them?" can be useful if a patient becomes reluctant to express their anxieties. It can also be appropriate not always to give an opinion when a patient asks for advice, but to reflect the question back to the patient by asking what he or she thinks would be for the best.

Counselling skills are also needed with asthma patients when there may be problems of non-compliance. Such problems will be more readily picked up if we can encourage an open, two-way dialogue.

To complete the consultation and to confirm that we have understood the patient and that he or she has understood us, it is useful to recap on the main points before giving guidelines for review.

From the professional's own position, clear, concise and accurate record keeping is essential for providing everyone involved with information for future consultation, as well as for legal protection. Finally, as part of a team, we need to develop a consistency of approach that gives the patient confidence in all members of the team, whether they are based in the community or the hospital.

Jennifer King

Dr Jennifer King, D. Phil (Oxon), C Psychol, AFBPsS, is a Director of Opus Consulting, Bristol.

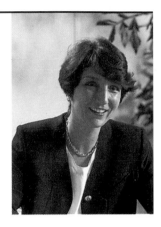

91
How can an unco-operative patient be managed during a consultation?

Understanding why a patient does not co-operate is the first step towards managing the problem. Patients come to the consultation with anxieties, beliefs and expectations which, research shows, have a strong impact on their decision to co-operate with professional advice. Anxiety itself can get in the way of the ability to listen and absorb information. Managing anxiety is therefore essential in gaining the patient's attention. Asking "Is there anything particularly bothering you about your asthma these days?" is helpful. This shows the patient that he or she is being heard and understood. It is also useful to explore particular beliefs the patient may hold about his or her asthma—"What do you believe brings on your asthma?"— "What do you think the blue inhaler is for?"—"How much of a worry is your asthma from day to day?" Questions like this make the consultation more of a two-way dialogue and promote greater co-operation.

Very resistant patients will often stay silent throughout the consultation. The temptation is to keep talking, firing advice and information at them in the hope that something will be absorbed. This is like shooting stray bullets, most of which will miss the mark. Silence—if prolonged—needs to be confronted. "You're very quiet—tell me what's on your mind" is a good open-ended approach. (Closed questions like "Is something bothering you?" may just provoke a straight "No" reply.) If resistance continues, there are various options.

- Acknowledge the resistance and continue with some very selective advice— emphasising the really important points.
- Be honest and direct: "The only way I can help you is if we are both involved in the conversation. I could continue to advise you but I do not know whether my advice is suiting you. What do you think?"
- Acknowledge the resistance and present a list of treatment options— "You can do a, b or c—a will have this effect; b this effect and c . . . etc.— which of these would suit you best?"

In general, make your advice very specific, with a time-scale if necessary. ("Let's agree that by the end of this month you will have done x"). Then agree a follow-up and also agree what should happen if the advice is not or cannot be followed for any reason ("If you find you cannot stick to it, what will you do?") Give the responsibility to the patient, but maintain a genuine attitude of support. Above all, do not "over care" about whether or not the patient is co-operating—this will stress you as well as the patient, who will feel pressured. Explore and listen to the patient's beliefs and views, acknowledge feelings and concerns, state your view, present options and reach some agreement—even if only on one small area to start with. Work to build trust, and co-operation will follow more easily.

Michael Hyland

Professor Michael Hyland, PhD, C Psychol, is
Professor of Health Psychology at the University
of Plymouth.

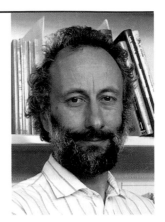

92
What is the value of quality of life assessment in asthma management?

"Assess before you intervene" is as good a piece of advice as any. Quality of life assessment is just one of several different types of assessment which can be used in asthma management. Quality of life refers to the patient's own subjective understanding of the impact of asthma and asthma treatment. It includes the physical limitations and the emotional upset, as well as the worries caused by asthma. It includes the burden caused by treatment, the cost and inconvenience.

The simplest way to measure quality of life is to ask patients how asthma affects them, and this can be done in the course of an interview. However, there are so many different ways that asthma affects patients—each patient is unique—that it is easy to miss important aspects of quality of life deficit from an interview alone. An alternative method, therefore, is to use a questionnaire, either alone or, as I would recommend, as a pre-interview guide for the consultation itself. Several different quality of life questionnaires are freely available to practising clinicians. The "Living with Asthma Questionnaire", "The St George's Respiratory Questionnaire", and the "Asthma Quality of Life Questionnaire" are all instruments that were developed originally as outcome measures in clinical trials. Each of these has advantages and disadvantages. The "Asthma Bother Profile" was developed as a pre-interview assessment tool and focuses primarily on the emotional impact of asthma. However, any of these instruments can be   195 used as a pre-interview assessment, and when used as such they do not need to be scored. Simply scanning down the patient's responses will give the health professional a good picture of how the patient is being affected by his or her asthma.

An important reason for using quality of life assessment is that it can give a very different picture compared with respiratory function testing. Some patients with good PEF report poor quality of life; and some with poor PEF report good quality of life. Although PEF and quality of life are correlated, the correlation is not large, because quality of life can be affected by many factors other than PEF. Asthma care should not simply be a matter of correcting the patient's respiratory function; it is also a matter of maximising the patient's quality of life.

One important finding from quality of life research is that although physical functioning can be improved by better physiological control of asthma, the emotional aspects of asthma are more readily changed by psychological factors. Asthma management involves both a physiological and psychological component—some patients report feeling better even though their respiratory function remains unchanged. Health professionals affect patients' psychology as well as their physiology. Quality of life assessment enables the health professional to detect psychological upset, as well as to measure its improvement following effective patient management.

Mike Townend

Dr Mike Townend, MB ChB (Hons), is a General Practitioner in Cockermouth, Cumbria.

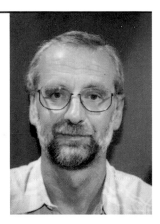

93

What advice should be given to an asthma patient who is about to go on holiday?

The advice needed by an asthma patient about to go on holiday will depend on the patient's mode of travel, destination and activities being undertaken on arrival, though some advice will be common to all. All asthmatic travellers need to ensure that they are carrying adequate supplies of medication plus additional supplies to allow for loss or for malfunctioning of inhalers. Preventive and relief medication should be carried with the traveller so as to be accessible when needed and preferably not all in the same bag or pocket in case of loss or theft. In aircraft, medication should be carried in hand baggage or on the person so as to prevent its arrival at a different destination from the traveller.

The asthmatic travelling to a destination remote from reliable emergency help should be instructed in the use of oral corticosteroids for an exacerbation and in the emergency use of high dose β_2 agonists via a large volume spacer which is more portable than a nebuliser and can be just as effective. A written self-management plan, ideally based on peak expiratory flow readings and a peak flow meter will complete the equipment needed.

During air travel some asthmatics' symptoms may be made worse by the poor quality or low humidity of the cabin air. Asthmatics should be advised to sit nearer to the front of the aircraft, where the quality of cabin air is better and the distance from the smoking area is greatest. If the holiday

197

involves crossing several time zones the timing of preventive medication will need to be adjusted, either gradually during the journey or by reconciling it with local time on arrival. Adjustments should preferably be made by shortening the gaps between doses rather than by prolonging them.

Other forms of travel may result in exposure to irritants, such as dust, temperature variations or tobacco smoke, or in enforced contact with allergens, such as animals. If the traveller is aware of his or her trigger factors problematic situations may be avoided or at least taken into account at the planning stage and medication adjusted to cope with them.

Holiday activities may vary from nightclubs and discos to skiing or high altitude mountaineering. Many activities will carry at least a potential risk to the asthmatic, ranging from smoky bars to physical exertion or breathing very cold air. Once again, the asthmatic with a good knowledge of his or her trigger factors and skill in self-management should be able to cope with these risks. Exercise-induced asthma, for example, may be dealt with by optimising the regular management and control, by using prophylactic β_2 agonist inhalation prior to exertion or by adding a long acting β_2 agonist drug to the regime, or by any combination of these.

Melinda Letts

Melinda Letts, BA Hons (Oxon), MIMGT, is Chief
Executive of the National Asthma Campaign.

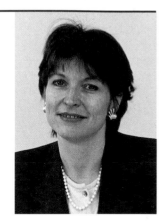

94
What are the questions asthma patients most often ask the Asthma Helpline?

The National Asthma Campaign has been running the Asthma Helpline since 1990. The Helpline offers independent information, advice, support and counselling to people with asthma and their carers. Staffed by asthma nurse specialists, all with varied clinical backgrounds and additional listening and counselling skills, it is open from Monday to Friday 9 am to 9 pm.

Advice given by the Helpline is based on the British Guidelines on Asthma Management, tailored to suit individual needs. The nurses consider the level of understanding of the caller and also how comfortable or distressed they may be with the information that they have received. Where appropriate this information is reinforced with National Asthma Campaign booklets and factsheets which are sent out the same day. The nurses on the Helpline also offer the caller confidentiality, anonymity, time and non-judgemental advice.

Daily the Helpline receives questions such as: "Why do I need a peak flow meter?" "Are there any long-term side effects to the medication?" "I am allergic to house dust mite: should I buy a new vacuum cleaner?" "What about complementary therapies to treat asthma?" Very often callers are parents of children with asthma. Common questions include: "What effects will steroids have on my child?" "Should I get rid of the cat?" "My child hasn't had an attack for a month so can I stop the medication?" "My son is 199 not allowed to have his inhaler with him in school. What can I do about it?" The Helpline nurses know the facts and can deliver the appropriate information to the caller.

Very often there is a hidden agenda in the question that the trained asthma nurse specialist must pick up and address as well. "What sort of nebuliser can I buy my daughter for Christmas?" begs information from the caller. "Why does she need a nebuliser?" "What is her current treatment and could it be altered to give more beneficial effects, thus negating the need for a nebuliser?" Through considered and informed communication, the root of the problem emerges and the parent can then make a decision based on the advice.

Many common questions require expansive answers. The patient who asks: "I am pregnant. Is it safe to take my asthma medication?" or "Should I have my child allergy tested?" may be hoping to gain information before an appointment with their GP, looking for reassurance, needing a chance to talk at ease about their condition or checking that the information they received from their doctor or nurse is consistent with that offered by asthma specialists. Facts and figures are not enough.

In 1995 the Asthma Helpline answered 17,179 calls and the most frequent questions concerned medication. 41% of callers asked for advice on their treatments, 36% wanted to know about asthma generally, 22% talked about self-management and peak flow and 18% asked about drug devices. The remainder covered changes in symptoms and the effects of the indoor environment.

Susan Kay

Susan Kay, MA, MCIMDip M, MICFM, is Acting Chief Executive of the British Lung Foundation.

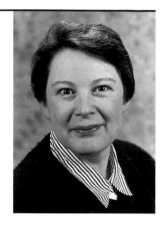

95
How do you evaluate the success of patient leaflets?

All organisations providing information to health professionals or the general public need to know that the information they produce is not simply accurate, but useful and relevant to the reader; it also helps if the material is in an easy-to-understand format. One method of assessment is simply by looking at the numbers requested and the repeat orders, especially from health professionals. The British Lung Foundation sends out some **30,000** leaflets every month, many as repeat orders from busy health professionals in GP surgeries or chest clinics.

To the consultant, GP or nurse, the value of good patient information in a simple leaflet is that the patient can take it away with them. Then, if the patient cannot always remember what was said about their particular condition, they can read about it at home in their own time. Of even more benefit is the fact that family members can also read about the condition and its signs and symptoms. This can help the family to understand the problem and come to terms with the practical aspects, such as impact on quality of life or potential side effects of treatment.

All organisations which publish patient information leaflets are constantly looking at how to expand the range to meet the needs of patients. New leaflets are developed from a range of requests—for example, following patient feedback questions from the British Lung Foundation's Breathe Easy Club or concerns expressed to doctors. In this category the British 201

Lung Foundation recently published a new leaflet on corticosteroid treatment for asthma to allay patient fears. GPs, in particular, had expressed views that patients were increasingly concerned about corticosteroid treatment. This view was confirmed following publication. From just one very small piece in a national newspaper about the leaflet more than 1500 requests were received.

Details of new treatments are also subjects for new leaflets and fact sheets, especially when the topic becomes "hot property" in the media. When the *Daily Mail* published an article on Lung Volume Reduction, the British Lung Foundation became inundated with people wanting to know more. The charity had to move quickly to solicit medical opinion and put together a balanced response that would answer the questions of a potentially vulnerable population.

What is certain is that patients are requesting more and more information and will quickly tell the provider if they do not feel it addresses the issues that concern them. This can only help to improve the range and quality of information provided on lung health issues.

Chapter 6

Policies and Organisation: Guidelines, protocols and roles

Christine Bucknall

Dr Christine E. Bucknall, MD, MRCGP, MRCP, is Career Registrar in the Department of Respiratory Medicine at Glasgow Royal Infirmary.

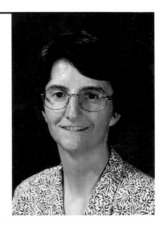

96
What outcome measures should be used to see if asthma management has been successful?

A good outcome for the individual with asthma will vary. Consequently, having some discussion with the individual about what you, as their health professional, and they are hoping to achieve will always be useful and sometimes very illuminating. In general, there are four sorts of outcome questions which will help measure the success of management.

The first of these questions is: "How much is this patient's asthma interfering with his or her life?" To answer this, think of identifying some activity and/or positive emotional state which applies when the patient is well—reviewing a self-completed quality of life questionnaire may help this search—and use this as a benchmark.

Second we should ask: "How well is the patient's asthma controlled?" This can be measured in terms of symptoms, peak flow variability and bronchodilator use. Everyone has their own favourite questions about symptoms, often including enquiry about sleep disturbance due to wheeze, morning chest tightness, cough and exercise-related wheeze. There are also validated measuring instruments available for measuring symptoms. Peak flow variability also provides information about asthma control, but remember that the faking of paper records is probably quite common. The degree of rescue bronchodilator use can be measured either by direct questioning or by prescription monitoring.

The third question to be asked is "How near to normal is the patient's lung function when he or she is stable?" The aim should be for values in the normal range, to ensure that the patient's airflow obstruction remains completely reversible. If there is any concern about this, then occasional assessment of best function with (increased doses of) inhaled or oral corticosteroids is indicated. In patients with partially irreversible airflow obstruction it is useful to aim to keep their stable lung function as near to their recent best as possible. This will prevent a gradual but progressive decline from passing unnoticed.

Our fourth question is: "Are side effects being minimised?" Aim to know about, and react to, short-term side effects of theophyllines, other bronchodilators and inhaled corticosteroids. Patients on oral cortico-steroids must be monitored for long-term side effects such as hypertension, diabetes and osteoporosis. Patients on high dose inhaled corticosteroids, perhaps because of intermittent courses of oral corticosteroids, may also merit monitoring for osteoporosis.

For small groups of patients, such as those within a practice, or attending a clinic, most of the measures described above can be aggregated, providing the data has been collected in a standard manner. The use of "percentage of best function" rather than "predicted" values for lung function in particular provides comparable data for groups containing varying proportions of patients with some irreversible air flow obstruction (for example, if data on groups of patients are being compared from year to year). This measure is also independent of treatment step. The "interference with lifestyle" measures are less easy to aggregate in a meaningful way if patient specific items rather than standard instruments have been used.

The same comments apply at a population level (district, hospital catchment or larger area), and in this context re-admission rates following hospitalisation for acute asthma may also be useful as an outcome measure, since recent evidence suggests they reflect the quality of discharge planning.

Ron Neville

Dr Ron Neville, MD, FRCGP, DRCOG, MBChB, is Principal in General Practice and Senior Lecturer and Director of Asthma at the Research Unit, Tayside Centre for General Practice, University of Dundee. He is Research Chairman of the GPs in Asthma Group.

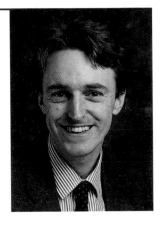

97
What methods and outcomes can be recommended and used to audit asthma care?

Audit is professionally satisfying, allows comparison of results between practices and clinics, and can identify "at risk" or problem groups of patients. There is no "gold standard" asthma outcome to compare with the HbA_1 in diabetes. British Guidelines on Asthma Management describe how asthma should be managed.

"Good care" should lead to:
- patients feeling better;
- appropriate use of preventative therapy; and
- appropriate use of health service resources.

Measurement of "good care" requires clinical assessment and review of case records, followed by repeat assessment and review. This principle of ongoing assessment and review underpins the various commonly used audit packages, such as the Tayside Stamp, the Action Asthma audit, the Jones Morbidity Index and the GRASSIC package.

"Good care" is associated with the following changes in the measures of process:
- more consultations with asthma trained practice nurses and fewer with general practitioners;
- more checking of inhaler technique and compliance; and
- more use of peak flow meters and self-management plans.

"Good care" is in turn associated with changes in patient well being and health service utilisation. A practice or clinic providing "good care" might expect:

- a reduced number of hospital admissions;
- fewer patient attendances at Accident and Emergency Departments due to asthma;
- fewer acute asthma attacks;
- fewer patients reporting symptoms such as night waking; and
- fewer patients with days lost from work, school or play.

To sum up, asthma audit is good for you, whether you are a patient or a healthcare professional.

Ruth Stearn

Ruth J.D. Stearn, RGN, SCM, NATC Dip in Asthma Care, is Lecturer/Practitioner Practice Nursing, Practice Nurse Assessor, Primary Care Audit Facilitator and a National Asthma Training Centre Regional Trainer.

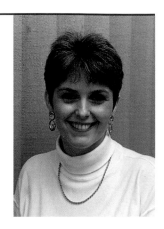

98
Does carrying out audit improve asthma care?

Asthma is well suited to audit because it is a common condition for which there are recognised, and therefore measurable, nursing and medical interventions. There are recommended treatments, as suggested by the British Guidelines on Asthma Management; issues of prescribing, such as reliever/preventer ratio; and also well described indicators of good or poor asthma control. Important aspects of investigation, diagnosis and patient education can also be included. Audit should therefore be seen as a vital part of the delivery of asthma care. It should be seen as a learning aid, an educational tool and a means of identifying problem areas.

Advances in the treatment and management of asthma are constantly under review, providing an opportunity to implement different approaches within various clinical settings and to monitor their effect in improving patient care. Changes implemented following audit are likely to benefit patients and there is a realistic potential for improvement.

Potential benefits of asthma audit include: improved awareness of the condition and its management; improved patient care through implementing change as a result of audit; improved job satisfaction for healthcare professionals; improved ability to justify treatment regimes; and improved team work. Asthma audit gives healthcare professionals the opportunity to take note of how they are delivering care at the present and to improve where care is sub-optimal.

Audit also allows health professionals to ascertain the prevalence of the disease within their practice population; to assess and recognise morbidity associated with the condition; to be accountable for the care they deliver; to identify problem areas, and to implement change to ensure the highest standard of asthma care delivery. Audit provides healthcare professionals with the opportunity to compare current asthma care with that of previous years or with other practices.

Acute asthma is an area where audit of current practice can lead to improved patient care. An exacerbation requiring emergency treatment or admission to hospital may be interpreted as a failure in the routine management of the condition. What were the events leading up to the exacerbation—could any of them have been prevented? Was there inadequate follow-up, inadequate use of prophylactic therapy, poor inhaler technique, poor patient education, or non-compliance with prescribed medication? Improved patient care can be a realistic outcome if deficiencies in care can be identified. Only by performing audit can any of these questions be answered.

The use of patient self-management plans can also be audited. Did the patient actually have a plan in the first instance? Were written guidelines given? Did the patient follow them? Did the patient contact medical personnel quickly enough and was the emergency treatment appropriate?

On completion of an audit it is important to look at achievements, emphasising what has gone well, what has been difficult, what has been learned and what are the next steps. Identifying causes of non-achievement is a useful exercise.

There must be agreement and understanding among the team if change is to be implemented. There must also be good reasons for making changes and it is essential that patients are going to benefit.

Performing asthma audit can lead to improvements in asthma care by ensuring that appropriate therapies via appropriate inhaler devices are prescribed, that regular review/follow-up is offered to asthma patients; and that issues of patient education are addressed in the asthma consultation. Poor asthma control can also be spotted by carrying out audit. Exacerbations/hospital admissions can be reduced and patient self-management can be encouraged.

Effective asthma audit allows participants to examine many aspects of their asthma management. The audit process should therefore be based on continuous assessment and improvement in the quality of health care given to people with asthma.

Christopher Langdon

Dr Christopher G. Langdon, BSc, LRCP, MRCS,
DRCOG, MRCGP, is a General Practitioner in
Maidenhead, Berkshire.

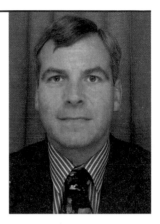

99
Why is asthma a unique condition in general practice?

Asthma is a very common condition which is undoubtedly increasing in
incidence. The number of asthmatics has risen dramatically over the last
decade, almost certainly in large part due to the willingness of GPs and
Practice Nurses to diagnose the condition. We are now prepared to make
a diagnosis of asthma in patients of any age, including in the young and
the very old. It is probable that at least 10% of the population suffers
from asthma. The great majority of these people are managed exclusively
in primary care.

What sets asthma aside from any other condition in medicine is that it is a
chronic, symptomatic condition which although seldom life threatening
can affect people of all ages, requires regular medication and causes enormous disruption to quality of life. Asthma attacks often involve many people
other than the patient. In children, attacks in the night will often disturb the
sleep of parents and siblings, leading to much lost productivity. At school,
peers and teachers are inevitably involved.

The diagnosis of asthma can be glaringly obvious or reached only after a
long process of consideration. Whatever else, a great deal of time needs to
be invested in the early stages on explanation and education. No matter
how asthma-wise we believe our patients to be, their education needs to be
reinforced at frequent and regular intervals by the GP and, perhaps more
importantly, the Asthma Nurse.

Medication involves a bewildering array of drugs and devices but the therapy can almost always be successfully tailored to the patient, so that people use a device with which they are comfortable and inhale a drug in which they are confident. The myths regarding the dangers of inhaled therapy are slowly disappearing and this can only increase patient confidence in their treatment.

Compliance, of course, remains a vital issue and there are numerous factors which influence the final patient adherence to our advice. It is said that patients actually do what we hope they do only 30% of the time, but this is also true of any other condition in medicine.

Asthmatics and their families have often been used to a life which most of us would find unacceptable. Now with better asthma care they are coming to understand that greatly improved quality of life is possible. It is often not until good control is achieved that patients fully understand what we are aiming at, and they are immensely grateful. In all but the very severest asthmatics this should be possible. I hope that our patients will accept nothing less as time goes on.

Every asthma patient must be treated as an individual, and many factors taken into consideration, before agreeing on a correct self-management plan. With time, enthusiasm and a desire to give our patients a normal lifestyle this surely is one of the most rewarding conditions to treat in general practice. Asthma is indeed, a unique condition.

Tony Crockett

Dr Antony Crockett, BM, DA, DRCOG, MRCGP, is a General Practitioner in Shrivenham, Oxfordshire and Clinical Assistant at the Asthma Clinic, Princess Margaret Hospital, Swindon, Wiltshire.

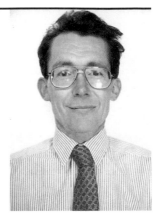

100
What should be included in an asthma protocol in general practice?

A protocol for asthma care is a plan for its management. Protocols are best devised by each practice and should involve all relevant members of the practice and primary health care teams. A protocol in general practice should include diagnosis, management, review/follow-up, and referrals.

Criteria for diagnosis should be agreed. Symptoms suggestive of asthma include recurrent wheeze or cough, especially at night, colds that "go to the chest", or exercise-induced symptoms. Suspicions should be higher in atopic patients or those with a family history of atopy. The diagnosis may involve the use of peak flow and symptom diaries, as well as trials of treatment, including a course of oral corticosteroids. All of these may be initiated by the GP or an experienced practice nurse (PN). Once the GP has made the diagnosis, it should be shared with the patient and clearly stated in the notes, whether computerised or manual. A register of all diagnosed patients should be kept and regularly updated.

The aims of management should be: to recognise asthma; to abolish symptoms; to prevent acute attacks; to maintain best possible lung function; to ensure best possible quality of life. To achieve these aims, a partnership with the patient must be made. The patient therefore needs: education; advice, support; time; and a listener. Advice on trigger avoidance must be relevant to each patient (take a careful history). Try to stop all patients smoking, either actively or passively. Give realistic, practical and individual 213 advice, and try to avoid inducing guilt. Follow or adapt the British Guidelines on Asthma Management. Agree guidelines on the use of peak flow meters, the use of self-management plans, the use of appropriate inhaler devices, including nebulisers, and when and how to step up or step down treatments. The whole practice team must be able to recognise acutely deteriorating asthma and agree how such patients can be quickly seen by the GP or PN.

For review and follow-up, the practice should agree which patients should be reviewed by the GP and which by the PN. This will depend on the skills and experience of the nurse and doctor, and on the severity and complexity of the patient's asthma. An example might be suspected asthma (PN or GP); diagnosis (GP); initial assessment (PN); regular review (PN); more complex or severe asthma (GP or experienced PN).

At each review, the health professional should: check (and adjust) inhaler technique; check peak flow readings and charts, if relevant; check compliance with management; make a detailed enquiry into symptoms and lifestyle; educate; listen; explain; check the self-management plan (does the patient know how and when to recognise deterioration, how and when to alter treatment, and how and when to call for help?).

All patients should be reviewed at least annually. Review more frequently if the asthma is more troublesome. Review all patients after any acute exacerbation, home visit, emergency nebulisation, Accident and Emergency Department attendance, hospital admission, or a rescue course of oral corticosteroids. This review may be hours or days after the event, depending on the circumstances.

External referral (from GP or PN to a hospital specialist) is needed: if there is diagnostic doubt; when asthma is difficult to control; before committing the patient to long-term oral corticosteroids or nebulisers; for occupational asthma; for patients with other complicating diseases.

Internal referral (from PN to GP) is needed: for any of the features requiring external referral; after a course of oral corticosteroids has begun; for persistent side effects from treatment; for concerns about a child's growth; if the patient or nurse is worried or requests referral. Internal referral (from GP to PN) should be the case for nearly all asthmatics, either on or after diagnosis.

In summary, protocols should be agreed and reviewed by the practice. Diagnostic criteria should be agreed. The PN and GP should share care, agreeing their respective responsibilities and roles. The practice should agree protocols for asthma management and follow-up, and for internal and external referrals. All protocols should be regularly reviewed, audited and altered if necessary.

David Price

Dr David Price, MA, MB BChir, MRCGP, DRCOG,
is a General Practitioner in Norwich.

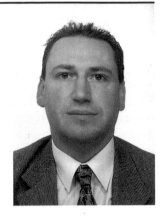

101
What are the cost implications of intensive primary care asthma management?

The computerised database of the Doctors' Independent Network of 800,000 patients suggests a 50% increase in asthma diagnosis over the period 1991 to 1995, outstripping increases in prevalence over that period. At the same time the percentage of patients with diagnosed asthma receiving inhaled corticosteroids has increased from 52% to 65%. This evidence suggests that those working in primary care are now more ready to diagnose asthma and are more aggressive in its management. However, one would expect resultant increases in asthma prescribing.

When looked at in my practice, asthma prescribing costs more than doubled over the period 1987 to 1994, from £39,706 to £89,040, principally due to increased inhaled corticosteroid prescribing, which rose from £14,734 to £53,640. This latter figure was some 35% above the local Family Health Services Authority (FHSA) average and we were asked to justify this high prescribing for asthma.

Increased prescribing costs, however, need to be set against a background of:
- increasing costs of asthma to society;
- increasing secondary care costs of asthma;
- increases in other primary care costs of asthma; and
- changes in outcome for the patients cared for.

Examining costs to society, the most obvious cost is certificated sick leave due to asthma. This increased from seven million working days in 1988 to 11 million in 1990. This may be a gross under-estimate as many patients with asthma either self-certificate or ask the doctor to certificate illnesses other than asthma. Accepting this at face value results in estimated costs of approximately £400 million in 1988 and £660 million in 1990. Furthermore, how do we put a price on more intangible costs, such as asthma deaths or effects of asthma morbidity.

Secondary care costs are also not insubstantial, with recorded admission rates for asthma increasing dramatically over the last 30 years. Estimated secondary care costs vary but the national figure is thought to be about £80 million per annum.

Primary care asthma costs can be broken down into drug costs, GP and practice nurse consultation costs, and other costs such as inappropriate antibiotic and cough suppressant prescribing.

It is clearly important to consider the whole picture and not just medication costs when looking at asthma treatment costs. When this was done in my practice, we found that alongside increased prescribing costs there were substantial improvements in care costs:

- Out of hours calls fell by 55% for asthmatics registered from 1990 to 1994.
- Surgery attendances with the nurse and GP fell 37% for the same group.
- Recorded exacerbations fell 25% in the same group.
- Bronchodilator prescribing fell per asthmatic by 45% from 1987 to 1994.
- Hospital admissions fell 43% to 10% of the local average between 1987 and 1994.
- Hospital outpatient attendances fell 65% over this period to 10% of the local average.

Whilst it is difficult to compare costs between practices, we have compared costs of our respiratory prescribing and hospital care with those of the local FHSA average. Inhaled corticosteroid prescribing cost 35% more, other respiratory drugs cost 15% less; but our secondary care costs were substantially less, resulting in our practice costing £23,000 less overall. This saving is more than the cost of a full-time asthma nurse and I would argue shows that intensive primary care asthma management is cost-effective.

Martyn Partridge

Dr Martyn R. Partridge, MD, FRCP, is Consultant
Physician at Whipps Cross Hospital, London. He
is Chief Medical Adviser to the National Asthma
Campaign.

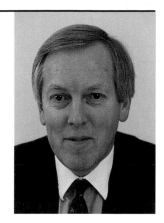

102
What should be included in an A&E protocol for managing asthma?

There are estimated to be three million people with asthma in the United
Kingdom, and 110,000 admissions to hospital because of asthma each year.
Presumably a significantly higher number attend Accident and Emergency
(A&E) Departments because of asthma, receive treatment and are allowed
home, but there are no national figures available for these attendances. In
the United States, it was estimated that in one hospital six per cent of all
emergency room attendances were because of asthma.

A recent National Asthma Census of Emergency Departments showed
that half of those attending were aged under 15 years of age, and a quarter
of those attending were aged five years or less. Sixty-two per cent of the
pre-school-age children were admitted, but thirty-nine per cent of the
adults who attended the A&E Department with asthma were also
admitted. Thirty per cent of those attending the A&E Department
with asthma had had no contact with their GP for at least a month prior
to attendance, and not all of the attendances for asthma were acute since
it was found that many of the adults had been kept awake for several
nights prior to attendance. A third of those attending the A&E
Department had been admitted to hospital in the previous 12 months, and
a quarter had attended the A&E Department in the previous three
months. Patients attending A&E Departments are therefore probably
high risk patients.

217

The British Guidelines on Asthma Management contain detailed advice on the management of adults and children presenting with acute severe asthma. They include advice regarding the assessment of severity, admission criteria and advice on what should be done before the patient returns home. The guidelines also contain detailed advice as to the correct management of asthma in A&E Departments. This medical information, which has been summarised on a chart, should form the basis of any A&E Department protocol.

Studies undertaken into the efficacy of such guidelines have shown improved outcomes associated with the introduction of the guidelines into A&E Departments. This is true especially when the guidelines for acute severe asthma are incorporated into record keeping; so that an observation prompts the correct line of management. A study of paediatric admissions from an A&E Department has also suggested benefit (in terms of reduced admission rates and safe discharge) following the use of either a more senior member of staff to assess those attending, or after an intensive training of more junior staff. Another study has shown that use of peak flow readings in children old enough to use them can also permit the safe discharge of some children if guidelines are adopted.

Purchasing authorities should therefore require the following from hospitals running A&E Departments:

- Evidence that the British Guidelines on Asthma Management are being implemented, and that there is adequate training of junior staff, implementation of guidelines into record keeping where appropriate, and regular audit of care.
- Realisation of the high risk nature of many of those attending with asthma. Repetitive attenders should be identified and referred to specialist clinics, either in hospital or in the community. There should be a set procedure to ensure that primary care asthma specialists are kept informed of attendances of their patients, if necessary by telephone or fax. Attending patients should be given written advice to see their GP urgently for follow-up.
- Whilst the A&E Department may not be the ideal venue for education, it may be the only opportunity, and written information personalised to that patient should be made available and opportunities to provide more information should be considered, such as the showing of video tapes on asthma during nebulisation.
- Patients being discharged from an A&E Department should be given written information about their medication.

Jill Logan

Jill Logan, RGN, NATC Dip in Asthma Care, is a Practice Nurse in Fife, Scotland and a National Asthma Training Centre Regional Trainer.

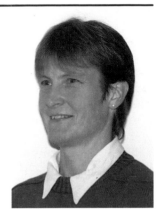

103
How can continuity of care be ensured between hospital and general practice for the adult asthmatic?

Some adult asthmatic patients require not only primary care but also secondary care. Communication is central to most issues in team-working and if not addressed can lead to a less than ideal situation in which the patient suffers most.

The patients who require secondary care are those who are difficult to manage in primary care, i.e. patients with occupational asthma, asthmatics who are dependent on oral corticosteroids and those who are poorly controlled. Patients attend secondary care as in-patients, and at Accident and Emergency (A&E) and Outpatient Departments.

As with any chronic condition, the continuity of care must be continually assessed in order to enable the patient to receive the best possible service. To rely solely on the patient relating "relevant" information from one department to another would prove unsatisfactory. Many patients undergo stress when attending hospital departments and as a consequence facts may become confused, resulting in information being neither correct nor beneficial.

In a secondary care setting, patients must have the opportunity to air their worries, concerns and questions. The staff who deliver and prescribe care must be up to date with current asthma guidelines and be seen to carry out care at this level. The same basic messages must be repeated by all health

219

professionals, and core information should ideally be written down and constantly updated.

Secondary care can be given without knowledge of the general practitioner. Written information is therefore essential in order to provide the patient with continuity of care. Examples of useful written information between primary and secondary care include the patient's current asthma therapy (and guidance as to whether he or she adheres to the currently prescribed regime), the patient's current inhaler device (especially if change has been instigated), recent peak flow (PEF) recordings (noting "best ever" when applicable) and if and when follow-up has been arranged.

Written information must be in a form that the patient can easily interpret and with which he or she will feel a sense of ownership. If it is not read by all care givers and then discussed with the patient, it is of little or no value. A co-operation card carried by the patient can continually be added to by both primary and secondary care health professionals and should also allow space for the patient's own queries, thoughts and feelings.

The importance of relaying this information between hospital and general practice must be stressed to the patient. However, it is not solely the patient's responsibility to relay this information and ideally it should be faxed between hospital and general practice at the time of discharge or A&E/Outpatient attendance. This would ensure less chance of the patient being "lost" in the follow-up system of the primary care setting.

The adult asthmatic's quality of life is at the centre of the issue of continuity of care. The best possible communication between care givers and patients, and between primary and secondary care teams, should improve overall patient care and patient morbidity.

John Haughney

Dr John Haughney, MB, ChB, MRCGP, DRCOG, is a General Practitioner at Calderwood, East Kilbride, Glasgow, Coordinator of the Lanarkshire Asthma Project and a member of the Asthma Working Party, Scottish Intercollegiate Guidelines Network.

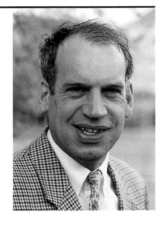

104

What is the role of the nurse in asthma care in general practice? The GP's view.

Nurses with specialist training are gaining increasing acceptance and popularity. This development has been encouraged by changes in General Practitioners' contracts, the demands of chronic disease management programmes, acknowledgement of the role of the nurse as clinician and educator and the availability of formal higher level training.

Asthma is a condition which can and should be managed principally in the community. Primary care nurses have the opportunity to be involved in the management of asthma sufferers at varying levels. Education and training centres and their awards of diplomas as markers of expertise have led to the development of a nurse-run primary care asthma service. At this highest level of involvement, the nurse can be responsible for the structure of the clinic, patient assessment and follow-up, development of treatment plans, telephone advice and on-going education.

Nurses who work in general practice have often to confront traditional views, even prejudices, about their role. Some patients identify a nurse as "a doctor's helper", even confusing nursing staff with administrative staff. Some doctors feel threatened by a perceived loss of their position. Most patients have their fears allayed as the new relationship between patient and nurse as clinician develops. The introduction of guidelines or practice-based protocols, as agreed between all health professionals, helps to clarify the   221 roles of each team member. Clearly defined responsibilities can help reduce misunderstandings. A nurse must not be asked, and should refuse to perform, a task for which she does not feel properly trained.

The successful organisation of a nurse-run clinic requires:
- a practice register of asthma patients;
- an effective recording system;
- an enthusiastic, trained nurse;
- an enthusiastic doctor;
- the support of the whole primary health care team;
- a practice guideline for asthma management.

Prior to developing an appropriate depth of training and knowledge, nurses may be involved in the practice asthma service with less ultimate responsibility. In this case, the patient will see a doctor at each visit. The nurse's role might include demonstrating and checking inhaler technique, routine data collection (including peak flow reading) and offering education and support.

A ladder of asthma knowledge has been described and should be employed. This is an attempt to avoid overwhelming the patient with too much information at once. Education and reinforcement are the cornerstones of good asthma management.

For the future, a natural progression would see suitably qualified nurses prescribing for asthma. This, however, will require a still greater depth of training, a willingness to accept greater responsibility for outcome and changes in current legislation.

The training and structure of their development as "asthma nurses" can also be utilised in other areas. Their qualities of enthusiasm, commitment and understanding enhance a primary care service.

June Roberts

June Roberts, SRN, DIP HE (PN), NATC Dip in
Asthma Care, is a Practice Nurse Manager/
Trainer in Salford, Greater Manchester and
a National Asthma Training Centre
Regional Trainer.

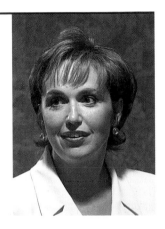

105
What is the role of the nurse in asthma care in general practice? The nurse's view.

The role of the nurse in asthma care in general practice depends on partnerships, co-operation and teamwork. The GP and Practice Nurse, alongside other members of the primary health care team, should work together to organise a structured programme of asthma care to benefit the practice population. The roles of the team members are complementary. Each is to be valued. Appropriately trained nurses working in general practice are well placed to take a lead role in improving the management of asthma.

The nurse's role in asthma care is as diverse as are individual practices. Many factors influence the amount of involvement—time, cost, medical support. Most important is the depth of the individual nurse's skill and knowledge. To work with any degree of autonomy the nurse requires specialist training, support from medical colleagues, experience of working with asthma patients and a high level of motivation. The nurse-led asthma clinic can enhance the effectiveness of asthma care.

Increasing involvement in asthma care presents a challenge to the nurse. There is added accountability to mirror the increase in professional responsibility. Also an implicit requirement to keep up to date with current trends in treatment and management. The nurse's role should include the dissemination of knowledge to other members of the team, communicating and sharing information. On a personal level, increased involvement of the

223

nurse in asthma care gives great professional satisfaction and mental stimulation. We can make patients feel better and that is rewarding!

The extent of the nurse's role in asthma care varies from practice to practice. There is a spectrum of involvement from minimal level to nurse-led asthma clinics. Expansion of the role of the nurse has to be negotiated and agreed with GP colleagues. By way of agreed practice protocols, with training and support, the nurse's role can be slowly expanded in the areas of: assessment and diagnosis; treatment; review and follow-up; patient education; communication; and audit.

In the area of assessment and diagnosis, the nurse's role can involve taking a detailed history and performing tests of lung function, including reversibility and exercise tests, and teaching the use of a peak flow meter and symptom diary for recording at home.

The nurse can play an important part in the implementation of national and local guidelines for treatment and management. Other treatment roles can include the selection and demonstration of inhaler devices and the checking of inhaler technique. The nurse might also be the first health professional to see patients in an emergency.

Regular review and follow-up roles for the nurse can include monitoring the patient's response to treatment, identifying poor control, giving telephone advice and establishing referral procedures.

It is perhaps in the area of patient education that the nurse can be most effective. Major contributions include: establishing what the patient already knows; exploring health beliefs; making patient education flexible, practical and specific; giving a little at a time; reinforcing at regular intervals; providing explanatory literature; negotiating self-management plans; backing up with written instructions; being an advocate for the patient.

Roles for the nurse in the areas of communication and interpersonal relationships can include: being a non-judgemental sounding board assessing patient compliance; exploring reasons for non-compliance; allowing the patient to express fears and worries; above all, listening. Finally, the nurse can take an active part in the audit cycle.

Asthma care has become one of the prime responsibilities for nurses in general practice. As asthma care has developed, the nurse's role has expanded. Today, nurses are developing expertise in the treatment and management of allergic disorders and chronic obstructive pulmonary disease to complement their existing skills. Nurses have excelled in providing a high standard of asthma care, and their role continues to grow.

Christine Fehrenbach

Christine Fehrenbach, RGN, NATC Dip in Asthma
Care, is Respiratory Nurse Specialist at
Portsmouth NHS Trust and a National Asthma
Training Centre Regional Trainer.

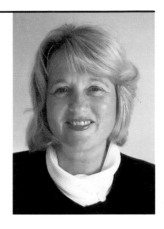

e. M. Fehrenbach.

106
What is the role of the asthma liaison nurse?

Successful asthma management results from putting together a large
number of components. Individually each component of asthma care has
only a relatively small effect. Together they can create a significant change
for the better. The essence of success is consistency of approach, together
with recognition of the enormous variation in the severity of the condition.
The role of the asthma liaison nurse is to facilitate a team approach during
the admission to hospital, the discharge back to the community and then in
the provision of shared care.

The acute attack can be successfully managed by evidence-based guidelines. The liaison nurse can be the thread weaving through the different
groups of health professionals involved—including non-respiratory teams
and Accident and Emergency personnel—to create an atmosphere of close
co-operation and consistency in communication. This collaboration helps
the various health professionals to recognise and respect each others' roles.
The ward nursing teams can have a respiratory link nurse scheme to enable
all departments to give updated care.

A good nurse–patient relationship can help the liaison nurse make use of
the window of opportunity for education and treatment review provided by
the acute attack. Patient perceptions are heightened during admission and
this makes it an excellent time to assess factors preceding the attack. A
reviewed negotiated treatment plan can be made on an individual basis. 225

Device selection is the responsibility of the nurse. Self-management plans should be given or amended at this time based on either symptoms or peak flow recordings.

Discharge planning should ensure that the asthmatic leaves hospital knowing when and where to seek help in the immediate future. An appropriate review can be arranged in general practice one week following discharge from hospital. The liaison nurse's role will have been to set up good communication channels through to primary care, for example using fax facilities, a practice nurse directory or a patient held co-operation card. The provision of a district-based asthma service helps in the development of these channels.

For the asthmatics who need secondary review a shared care service can be part of the liaison nurse's role. The aim should be that care should not be duplicated. Support can be given with the goal of improving self esteem, giving the asthmatic more control of his or her day-to-day life. In some districts a nebuliser service is run by the liaison nurse. The nurse can monitor and supervise the appropriateness and cost effectiveness of this provision. The service should include regular maintenance of the equipment and education in the care of it according to the British Guidelines on Asthma Management.

The asthma liaison nurse can act as a resource for other non-NHS agencies such as social workers, playgroups, residential homes and charitable organisations.

The nurse acting in the liaison role can thus uniquely work across boundaries to create better care for asthmatics. This improved care is the net result of combining all the individual components and, as is so often the case, the total result is greater than the sum of its individual parts.

Fiona Moss

Dr Fiona Moss, MD, MB BS, MRCP, is Associate Dean of Postgraduate Medicine, North Thames Health Authority, London.

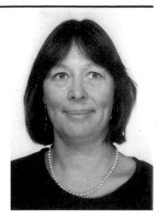

107
What is shared care? The consultant's view.

Finding the most appropriate treatment for someone troubled by asthma is an interactive process. Thus all asthma care is a process shared between patient and professional. Helping people to relate to their symptoms, to changes in airflow and the stability of asthma so that they can make adjustments to their treatment is a central part of the process of asthma care.

People with asthma may receive care from healthcare professionals based in either primary or secondary care or both. For many patients care is straightforward as they are able to receive care from primary care based doctors and nurse specialists and do not require referral to a secondary care based specialist or need admission to hospital. But for others the organisation of their care is not as simple. This may be because their asthma is particularly troublesome and they therefore need the attention of healthcare professionals based in both primary and secondary care; but for others care may be dispersed because of their circumstances; their jobs; or their life-styles. For all these people asthma care will need to be shared with more than one group of professionals.

Shared care begins with an acknowledgement that a patient needs to receive care from more than one source. Ideally all those who are partners in a shared care scheme—and this includes the patient—should be working with the same aims for the individual and with agreed criteria for changes in management or other action. Communication is an essential element of a shared care. All partners should have easy access to decisions made by others. Patient-held shared care cards—as used for maternity care—are an effective and cheap way of achieving this. Of course computers provide a way of linking primary and secondary care and allowing electronic passage of information. The advantage of the paper held record is that the patient has equal access to the information—and should be encouraged to record his or her own notes on the cards too.

Much lip service is paid to the notion of shared care. But simply for a patient to be seen sometimes in general practice and at others in the local chest clinic does not necessarily constitute shared care. Encouraging the development of genuine shared care and the use of effective patient held records will emphasise the role of the patient as a partner in care. Shared care should not be confined to care shared between primary and secondary care. For example the care of asthma in schoolchildren might be shared by the school nurse, the general practitioner, the parents and the child. And patient held records would contribute also to the care of students or anyone whose circumstances takes them away from home. Communicating well about asthma is central to all aspects of asthma care. So setting up shared care should not be too difficult.

Paul Stephenson

Dr Paul Stephenson, MA, BM BCh, DRCOG, DGM, MRCP, is a General Practitioner in Haverhill, Suffolk. He is Editor of "Asthma Care Today" and Chairman of Asthma 2000.

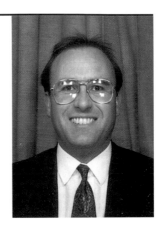

108

What is shared care? The GP's view.

"Shared care" is a frequently used term but one that tends to lose its fundamental meaning. I shall focus here on several important aspects of the team in relation to asthma. The "sharing" of asthma care can be on several levels: between primary and secondary care; within primary and within secondary care; and between professional carers and patients.

In the same way that midwives play a pivotal role in obstetrics, the asthma nurse plays a pivotal role in asthma care. Despite the fact that the role of the asthma nurse continues to evolve, the revolution that has occurred in primary care over the last five to six years (due to several factors but not least the advent of the National Asthma Training Centre and the explosion in numbers of Diploma-trained asthma nurses), has facilitated the shift of asthma care from the secondary to the primary care sector. Up to 95% of asthma care is now delivered solely in primary care.

The first level of sharing—between primary and secondary care— is thus probably only relevant to between 5 and 15% of the total asthma population. Of course, the asthma patients who do have dealings with secondary care (by the sheer nature of the fact that their disease is at the more severe end of the spectrum) constitute a disproportionate amount of the workload. Most GPs would agree that the initiation of "shared care" (i.e., recruiting secondary care expertise from a primary care setting) would occur in the following situations: uncertainty about the diagnosis of asthma; 229

patients not responding to standard asthma treatment—particularly those who look as though they need regular oral corticosteroids; occupational asthma; patients with a very considerable psycho-social aspect to their asthma, particular those with "brittle" disease; many of those patients requiring a hospital admission for asthma.

Since the management of asthma is now primary care led, a substantial number of those patients who are presented for "shared care" into the secondary care sector can be returned back to primary care as soon as secondary care has fulfilled its function. Good communication is essential here and much of it can be devolved to the respiratory specialist nurse in the hospital and the asthma nurse in primary care. Furthermore, good communication permits the setting of asthma guidelines within the district or region and increases the level of awareness in the locality.

The second level of shared care is what happens within primary or within secondary care. There is enough literature on communication within the primary health care team to fill a library! Yet, this is a major achievement of British General Practice. We have in place a highly effective and efficient primary health care system which is ideally placed to provide the optimum management of asthma within the community. The sharing of ideas between all the parties involved, can only lead to better, more individually tailored management for the patient. Similarly, secondary care "asthma clinic teams" are now commonplace, since they can provide a much more integrated approach to asthma management.

This leaves us with the third level of shared care—the sharing of care between healthcare professionals and patients. In primary care we are trained to manage asthma on a physical, psychological and social level. To provide optimum care, and to fulfil the ideal "shared care" model, four things are needed: first, knowledge—to a sufficiently high level that consistent advice is always given; second, application of knowledge; third, communication skills—in which primary care has a specific expertise, based on various consultation models which have helped us communicate better with patients, and fourth, time—good quality care takes time.

A major factor in the success of obstetrics shared care in this country is the hand-held patient record. This has obvious relevance to shared asthma care. Hand-held asthma records—containing all test results, peak flow charts, and comments from consultations and clinic attendances—would facilitate communication between all the healthcare professionals involved, and would remain in the patient's possession. As we enter into the 21st century, these records need not be on paper—the "asthma smart card", the size of a credit card, containing computer-held information on a patient's asthma, will be the tool for shared asthma care in the future.

Trisha Weller

Trisha Weller, MHS, RGN, NDN cert, DPSCHN
(PN), NATC Dip in Asthma Care, is National
Asthma Training Centre Regional Trainer for the
West Midlands.

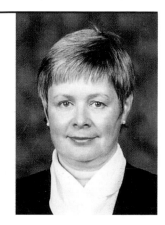

109
What is shared care? The nurse's view.

In the words of Dorothy L. Sayers: "A trouble shared is a trouble halved."
Traditionally, medical practitioners decided on patient care and treatment.
The nurse carried out the doctor's instructions in her "handmaiden" role,
while the patients did as they were bid. To question or fail to carry out
instruction, branded patients as non-compliant or deviant, while nurses
were likely to be severely reprimanded. The doctor was the pivotal part of
patient health care.

Fortunately, those days of dictated patient care are behind us and a
partnership or shared care is accepted as the way forward, with the patient
the key figure. Shared care is the division of care between the patient and
the health carer and the extended health care team, as well as lay persons
such as parents, siblings, school personnel and friends. The emphasis of
shared care is education and accurate information, allowing the individual
to choose whether to comply with instruction or not.

Patient expectations have increased and, correctly, patients now demand
information which will enable them to make choices. Responsibility has
shifted from the doctor to the patient but shared care will only succeed if
there is knowledge. The amount of knowledge that is required will vary
according to an individual's ability to understand.

Specific asthma education for the nurse, of a proven standard, is essential
for a high standard of asthma care. Poor or inaccurate information must be

avoided and discounted. A nurse may be a highly experienced asthma nurse specialist or may be a nurse with only minimal asthma knowledge. Recognition of the nurse's role in the asthma education chain is vital and will depend on his or her experience, knowledge and expertise. According to his or her own ability the nurse needs to gauge the correct level of information that the patient can absorb and to understand how that information can be imparted. The nurse needs to recognise when asthma control is poor and treatment is inadequate. Is the patient taking his or her prophylactic medication or is asthma control deteriorating? Can the patient use his or her inhaler? When should the nurse refer the patient back to the doctor? The role of the nurse in shared care is also about his or her own professional accountability.

Patients will vary in their degree of responsibility for their own health care, with parents taking responsibility for their children's health care as well as their own. The nurse's relationships with the parent and with the child are equally important. Elderly patients may sometimes find it difficult to have a deciding role in their own care and treatment, because they may not be used to questioning health professionals. The nature of general practice will enable the practice nurse to develop a relationship with a variety of patients. Many of these patients will regard the nurse not only as a health professional, but as an educator, counsellor, advocate and friend.

Shared care is a partnership which should enable the patient to take responsibility for his or her health and health outcomes. A symptom-free lifestyle with no restrictions is the aim of successful shared care.

James Friend

Dr James Friend, MA, MB, FRCP Ed, is
Consultant, Thoracic Medicine at Aberdeen
Royal Infirmary and Clinical Reader in Medicine at
Aberdeen University. He is Chairman of the
Asthma Working Party, Scottish Intercollegiate
Guideline Network.

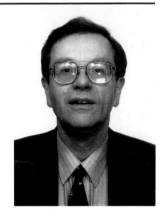

110
Should international, national or local asthma guidelines be followed?

Guidelines cause a variety of reactions; they are either respected, derided or
ignored. Guidelines now run the risk of multiplying into almost every field
of clinical practice, with doctors and nurses becoming buried in volumes of
paper. As far as asthma is concerned, we now have international guidelines
and, in the UK, the British Guidelines for Asthma Management. In
addition, local guidelines have been published, including the GP guidelines
for the North-East of England and the hospital guidelines for Scotland, and
others are in preparation. There are also many local asthma protocols,
ranging from area protocols to those agreed for a single hospital or general
practice setting. All this diversity could be confusing; what achieves the best
results for people with asthma?

The ideal guideline is based on good evidence of the highest scientific
quality, derived from a comprehensive literature search and grading the
quality of the evidence. The best evidence derives from properly conducted
controlled clinical trials, but at present only a minority of the evidence in
current guidelines is of this quality. Much is of GOBSAT quality—Good
Old Boys Sitting At Table!

It is not easy to write guidelines, but even harder to put them into
practice. If those who are expected to use guidelines play no part in their
development, they will see them as having been imposed by people who
have no real understanding of the "real world" in which the doctor or nurse   233

is working. For instance, the care of asthma in an inner city is very different from that in a rural area where the nearest hospital is 80 miles away and the GP lives in the village. Guidelines can indeed improve the quality of clinical practice, but they are much more likely to be effective if they take account of local circumstances, are disseminated by an active educational intervention, and if they incorporate the use of patient-specific reminders at the times when decisions are made.

Early guidelines perhaps had an inevitable emphasis on drug therapy for asthma, but giving the right drug treatment is only a part of asthma care. Major differences in outcome arise from improvements in the process of care—the way in which services for people with asthma are organised and delivered. Examples include methods of patient education, hospital discharge procedure and GP follow-up policies. The evidence base for guidelines in such areas is sparse. The writing of local guidelines, and their development into local protocols by local groups involving nurses, doctors, patients and others, offers a real opportunity for very local direct involvement, for clinical audit and for high-quality local research.

International and national guidelines, if fully evidence-based are a vital foundation for local guidelines and protocols. Local, multi-disciplinary groups need to adapt these to local circumstances if individual people with asthma are to benefit.

Ann Dawson

Dr Ann Dawson, BA (Hons), MSc, MRCP, is
Senior Medical Officer with the Health Care
Directorate, NHS Executive, London.

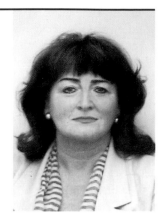

111
What should be included in national asthma policies?

The aim of national public health policy is to keep asthma sufferers free of
symptoms and able to lead as normal a life as possible. Sufferers need to
know their individual trigger factors and how to avoid them, and the
practical steps and medicines they should take to control their symptoms.
The objective is to enable people with asthma to manage their own condition as effectively as possible, with help and advice from their doctor,
specialist nurse and others in the primary care team.

The Department of Health has provided a national framework for the
provision of general medical services for asthma in its Chronic Disease
Management Programme (CDMP), which was introduced in 1993. Over
90 per cent of general practitioners in England are now participating.

The CDMP requires participating practitioners to set up an organised
programme for the care of patients with asthma, with clearly understood
arrangements for any shared care with the secondary sector. Within the
programme they should:
- keep a register of all patients with asthma;
- ensure systematic call and recall of patients;
- ensure that all newly diagnosed patients with asthma, and their carers
  when appropriate, receive relevant education and advice;
- in association with the patient, prepare an individual management plan,
  which includes advice on how to record and interpret peak flow readings; 235

- ensure that all established patients, and where appropriate their carers, receive relevant continuing education, including supervision of inhaler technique if appropriate;
- carry out regular medical reviews (generally every six months) of the patient, including peak flows and all other relevant investigations, to establish the degree of severity of the condition and any associated complications;
- ensure that all health care professionals concerned with the care of patients with asthma are appropriately trained and receive continuing education;
- refer patients to other services as necessary;
- maintain adequate patient records; and
- carry out clinical audit of the care of patients with asthma.

General practitioners participating in the CDMP have to submit an annual report to the health authority detailing the number of patients with asthma by age and sex; and the number of those patients who have (a) received regular prophylactic medication for their asthma, (b) had their peak flows measured within the past year, and (c) been admitted to hospital as a consequence of their asthma.

The CDMP sets out how primary care for asthma should be provided. The Department of Health has also commended to the NHS the British Thoracic Society's revised guidelines—the British Guidelines on the Management of Asthma—which include advice on how patients should manage their own condition. This is the key to achieving a better quality of life for people with asthma.

Mike Pearson

Dr Mike Pearson, MA, MB BChir, FRCP, is
Consultant Respiratory Physician at Aintree
Chest Centre, Liverpool and Associate Director
of the Research Unit of the Royal College of
Physicians.

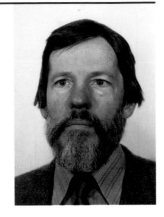

112
How can clinical trials of asthma therapy be critically appraised?

New therapy should be compared either with a placebo or, if it is not ethical
to withhold an established treatment, with that established treatment. Most
placebo trials show benefit from the placebo (probably due to better
compliance during the study), so a new treatment has to better the placebo
result statistically and, more importantly, should be shown to do so in more
than one clinical trial.

Randomised control trials (RCT) are performed blind (i.e., neither
patient nor doctor knows which is the active or the placebo drug), and
patients who meet the entry criteria should have been allocated randomly to
the placebo or active arms of the study. Results should be presented on an
"intention to treat' basis, with all those who began in the trial being
included in the analysis.

An alternative is to treat the same patients with both new and placebo (or
established drug) preparations sequentially but with the order randomised.
This has the advantage of each patient acting as his or her own control, but
results may be difficult to interpret if there is a carry-over effect from the first
to the second treatment periods.

Asthma varies from a mild exercise-induced wheeze to a severe incapa-
citating condition. The variation occurs between different persons and also
within the same person. Trials need to show how mildly or severely the
subjects were affected, and whether they were stable or unstable, before the   237

results can be extrapolated to other patients. Results in a group with severe unstable asthma may not be relevant in mild and stable asthma.

Many studies use improvement in either the forced expiratory volume in the first second of inspiration (FEV_1) or peak flow (PEF) to signify success. If changes are large—for example, 25% improvement overall—there is little doubt about benefit. When changes are small—for example, 5–10% overall—it is difficult to know if the benefits are real and even harder whether the benefits are worthwhile. Most patients may have felt better, but some may not. Statistical tests differentiate between a true positive result and findings that could have arisen by chance. The statistical significance is often expressed as a p value:

$p < 0.05$	Likely to occur by chance once in 20 trials.	Possibly significant.
$p < 0.01$	Likely to occur by chance once in 100 trials.	Probably significant.
$p < 0.001$	Likely to occur by chance once in 1000 trials.	Very significant.

Studies that only have values of p equals 0.05 should be read cautiously and only accepted when there are other data to confirm the findings.

The only way of knowing if small changes are worthwhile is to ask the subjects. Thus many studies also record asthma symptoms and, more recently, the "quality of life". If all the different measurements point in the same direction, then a greater degree of confidence should be placed in the results.

In general, the more patients included and the longer the period of study, then the more likely are the results to be true. Short studies of a few weeks could be confounded by seasonal effects, and small studies could by chance have included atypical subjects. The statistical analysis should make allowance for this, but in practice will often not do so. It is perhaps best always to look for more than one study from different centres before reaching conclusions.

Many asthma treatment studies are sponsored by pharmaceutical companies. In general, their involvement has been extremely ethical and the standards they work to are very high, and the published results have been shown to be valid over time. Again, the best way of removing the doubts about bias is to compare multiple studies from different centres.

Rashmi Shah

Dr Rashmi R. Shah, BSc (Hons), MBBS (Lon), MD (Lon), FRCP (Edin), FFPM (UK), is Senior Medical Officer at the New Chemical Entities Unit, Licensing Division, Medicines Control Agency, London.

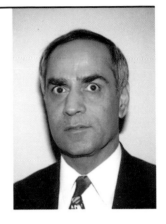

113
What is the role of the Medicines Control Agency?

The pharmaceutical sector in the UK is regulated by the Licensing Authority (LA) which consists of six designated Government Ministers. The Medicines Control Agency (the MCA) is the executive arm of the Licensing Authority and regulates all aspects of human medicinal products in the UK.

The primary purpose of the MCA is to safeguard public health by ensuring that human medicines available in the UK are made to the highest standards of quality and are evaluated for safety and efficacy before and after they are approved and licensed for sale and supply. The MCA is not concerned with the actual clinical use of the drug/product, which is a matter for the clinical judgement of the physicians.

The legislative powers and the parameters within which to regulate the pharmaceuticals flow from The Medicines Act, 1968, various statutory instruments and an array of Directives from the European Union (EU). The Agency represents UK interests in all pharmaceutical activities at the EU level.

The Agency is divided into five Divisions, three of which are concerned directly with quality, safety and efficacy. The Licensing Division of the MCA receives applications for clinical trials in patients and for product licences. The application may relate to a new chemical entity or a previously licensed drug for a new indication, dose schedule or formulation. Appli-

239

cations are also received for "copies" of drugs already licensed (generic products). After validation, the data supporting each application are assessed by MCA professional assessors specialising in toxicology, pharmaceutics and clinical medicine. For generic products, particular attention is given to ensure that the product is essentially similar and therapeutically equivalent to the one already on the market.

The LA/MCA frequently takes independent expert advice on matters relating to safety, quality and efficacy from advisory bodies. Perhaps the best known of these advisory committees is the Committee on Safety of Medicines. Its members are appointed by Ministers and do not include any of the MCA staff.

Following a decision to grant a licence, the Summary of Product Characteristics (SPC) is agreed with the applicant. The SPC forms the basis of subsequent prescribing information and the Patient Information Leaflet. If a decision is made not to grant a licence, the applicant is given the reasons for this decision.

As soon as a product is marketed, the Post-licensing Division of the MCA monitors it for the pattern of adverse effects that may emerge following its administration to larger numbers of patients. Its risks and benefits are kept under surveillance. The Division ensures that the prescribing information satisfactorily reflects all available safety data, if necessary by amending as appropriate the SPC. Information affecting the safe and effective use of a medicine is communicated to the health professionals in the quarterly bulletin, "Current Problems in Pharmacovigilance", and in case of major safety concern, by letters from the Chairman of the Committee on Safety of Medicines. This Division also regulates the Patient Information Leaflets, promotion of a medicine (not only to the public but also to health professionals) and its legal status and method of supply— prescription only medicine (POM), pharmacy only (P) or general sales list (GSL).

Licences are required not only for marketing a product but also for its manufacture, wholesale distribution and import. Any number of various obligations may be attached to a licence. The Inspectorate and Enforcement Division regularly inspect UK manufacturing sites. Overseas manufacturing sites are inspected either by the UK Medicines Inspectors or, on their behalf, by the Inspectors in the country where manufacturing takes place. The UK Inspectors also maintain regular checks on the quality of the medicinal products and associated claims/literature on the retail shelves. Any defect or violation of obligations or terms of licence are appropriately dealt with, including immediate removal of the product from sale if necessary.

Bernard Taylor

Bernard Taylor, BSc, is the recently retired
Executive Chairman of Medeva plc.

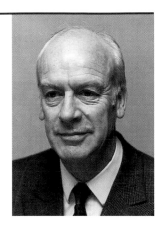

114
Will research based companies introduce new chemical entities for treating asthma if their market share and profits are reduced by generic companies who do not invest in research?

The cost of discovering and developing a new drug is now of the order of £200 million, a substantial investment for any company to undertake and one with a high probability of failure along the way. Without the protection afforded by patents, no company could consider such an investment. Any worthwhile discovery would be quickly copied and the originator would be unable to recoup his costs, let alone profit from his inventiveness.

A patent, however, does not confer a monopoly in perpetuity. The period of protection from copy products, or generics as they are called, is restricted to 20 years from discovery. This period is foreshortened by the time taken to develop and launch a new product worldwide, leaving about 8 to 10 years for a company to fully recover its costs—on the failures as well as the successes—and to make a reasonable return on its investment. The considerable commercial success of the innovative companies in the industry, and the remarkable advances they have made in treatments for most diseases, are testimony to the value of patents in a free enterprise society.

The drug discoveries of the 1960s and 1970s which revolutionised the prevention and treatment of asthma are now off-patent and cheaper, but high quality generics are making inroads in the market. However, the occasion of patent expiry on the original products has heralded a new era of 241 innovation which is benefiting patients. This time, rapid progress is being made in delivery systems, with generic companies competing with each other, and with the originators, to offer better systems of delivering drugs to the lungs.

But what of the future? In the pharmaceutical industry the future can be forecast to some degree because of the disclosure required by those seeking to patent their inventions and the long period required to develop a new product. What can be seen is that many of the most innovative companies are working on new approaches to asthma and a number of potential products are in the development pipelines. Pharmaceutical companies have to be aware of the commercial potential of their research and development investments. They have clearly recognised that there is still room for improvement in current treatments of asthma and that a substantial reward awaits those who succeed in finding solutions to remaining clinical problems.

One must conclude that current levels of patent protection are sufficient to encourage discovery of new treatments for asthma. Furthermore, that there is an important place for the generic companies, offering to patients older products, of good quality, and at favourable prices to the NHS.

Richard Sykes

Sir Richard Sykes, DSc, is Deputy Chairman and
Chief Executive of Glaxo Wellcome plc.

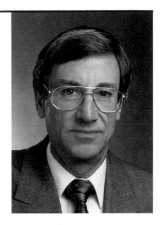

Richard B Sykes

115
Should an obligatory amount of industry profit be spent on education and training for health professionals?

As healthcare practice worldwide comes under increasing scrutiny and under increasing pressure to deliver value for money to its customers, both purchasers and providers of health care will look to the creation of new partnerships and alliances to ensure that the quality of delivery to the patient is not compromised. In developed countries, particularly in the USA and Western Europe, alliances are already being formed to create new initiatives that even 10 years ago would have seemed unlikely. Many of these focus around training and education—initially of professionals, and subsequently of patients—so that purchasers and providers can ensure that the maximum benefit is gained from medication.

Training is an integral part of the information cascade. Many medicines are not "simply swallowed" but are delivered direct to various sites in the body by sophisticated delivery systems. In respiratory medicine, for example, the correct use of inhaler devices is vital if patients are to benefit from their medication. It is obligatory for industry to invest in education and training in the use of its products if it wishes those products to be used effectively. Pharmaceutical companies are perforce *the* experts in their own medicines. Their obligation is to share their knowledge as widely as possible, among the professionals who are their partners, in order to ensure successful outcomes for the patients.

243

Glaxo Wellcome (Allen & Hanburys) have supported non-promotional educational training programmes in asthma care by working alongside organisations such as the National Asthma Training Centre, as well as substantial programmes with GPs and hospital specialists, to continue to further good asthma management initiatives. This alliance not only shows industry working in partnership with healthcare providers but also exemplifies its commitment to education and training.

Most research-based pharmaceutical companies already make a substantial investment in training and educating healthcare professionals. It is open to debate whether making such investment obligatory would increase total expenditure on training and education or ensure that available resources are targeted at areas of greatest need.